# A "Cute" Leukemia

## Rodney Curtis

---

### Read The Spirit Books
an imprint of
David Crumm Media, LLC
Canton, Michigan

For more information and further discussion, visit
*http://A-Cute-Leukemia.com*


Copyright © 2013 by Rodney Curtis
All Rights Reserved
ISBN:
April 1, 2013


Back Cover Photos:
  Top photo: Steve Perez
  Middle photo: Marci Curtis
  Bottom photo: J. Kyle Keener
All photos not otherwise credited were by the author


Cover art and design by
Rick Nease
www.RickNeaseArt.com


Published By
Read The Spirit Books
an imprint of
David Crumm Media, LLC
42015 Ford Rd., Suite 234
Canton, Michigan, USA


For information about customized editions, bulk purchases or permissions, contact David Crumm Media, LLC at info@DavidCrummMedia.com

# Contents

| | |
|---|---|
| Dedication: | vii |
| Bone Tired | 1 |
| The L-Word | 4 |
| Having Fun with Cancer | 7 |
| Blue Evening | 10 |
| Departure Terminal | 13 |
| No News is Good News | 16 |
| A Better Medicine | 20 |
| Chemo Sabes | 23 |
| Five Laps | 26 |
| Dear Nephew | 28 |
| Ode to an Egg Salad Sandwich | 31 |
| Half a Dozen Cupcakes | 33 |
| Hair Today, Gone Tomorrow | 37 |
| Bad News/Good (Detroit) News | 39 |
| Maybe a Wasp Took It | 42 |
| Clown Collage | 44 |
| This is ENN | 46 |
| In My Room | 52 |
| Dreadlocks for Love | 54 |
| Blimey, I'm in Rehab! | 55 |
| $#%t | 57 |
| Home | 60 |
| A Funraiser | 62 |
| Golden Bubbles and Silver Linings | 66 |
| Peter's Principles | 69 |
| Remission Accomplished | 72 |
| I Have a What the Size of a What, Where? | 75 |

| | |
|---|---|
| What Lies Ahead | 78 |
| Messing With the Messengers | 81 |
| Ends and Odds | 84 |
| Is the Patient In? | 86 |
| Blood Brothers | 87 |
| Next to Normal | 90 |
| To the Patient in Room 2603 | 93 |
| The Kids Are All Right | 95 |
| Far Too Much Time on My Hands | 98 |
| Dichotomy | 100 |
| An Occasional Little Schnuffle | 103 |
| A Breath of Fresh Hair | 106 |
| Born Again? | 109 |
| Tenth Floor | 112 |
| A Transplant Tutorial | 115 |
| My Main Marrow Man | 118 |
| Nadir and Me | 121 |
| It's not My-in, It Must be Urine | 123 |
| I Hear a Symphony | 127 |
| Our Hallucination | 129 |
| The Beginning of the NDE | 133 |
| You Asked About the Meaning of Life | 136 |
| Yoga, the Ultimate Sin | 139 |
| The Worst Christmas Card Ever | 142 |
| Honest Officer, It's the Ambien! | 144 |
| You Are My Person of the Year | 146 |
| Reports of My Death Are Greatly Exaggerated | 148 |
| My Nutter Brother | 149 |
| Day 100 | 151 |
| Cool or Creepy? | 154 |
| The Fighter | 156 |
| Tub Thai | 158 |
| The International Symbol for Embarrassment | 160 |
| Following My Heart | 162 |
| Mr. Compassion | 165 |
| Heavy Sigh | 167 |

| | |
|---|---|
| A Year and Today | 170 |
| Oh, Steroids | 172 |
| The Traumas of June | 174 |
| Interlacing Threads | 177 |
| Back in the Saddle (Again?) | 179 |
| Dumb & More Dummer | 182 |
| California Dreaming | 186 |
| Worldwind | 189 |
| These Are My People | 193 |
| This One's on the House | 196 |
| Here's to a Year | 198 |
| These Poor Corporations | 201 |
| Oh Christmas Tree | 205 |
| Tipoff | 208 |
| Hello Memories | 210 |
| Sweet Dreams | 213 |
| I Forgot to Write About Our Memory Test | 215 |
| Spring Eternally Hopes | 218 |
| These Moments | 220 |
| There's an App for That | 222 |
| If Only I Were a Poet | 224 |
| Relay | 225 |
| Graduation Day | 228 |
| About the Author | 230 |
| Colophon | 232 |

# A Note About the QR Codes In This Book

When I wrote this book, I did it on a computer like most reputable authors nowadays. I got it into my head that you shouldn't just have to read my dopey words, but if you felt like it, you could view some videos, see webpages and maybe even hear a sound or two. Since it was going to be an e-book, viewable on your iPad, Kindle, Nook, phone or some other fancy device, that wouldn't be a problem. Ahh, but if you are reading this book on paper, like people have done for almost six centuries since Johannes Gutenberg pressed a bunch of monks into retirement, then you'll see some of these crazy little square symbols. You've probably seen 'em before on ketchup bottles, mailing labels and maybe even certain fuzzy rodents of questionable repute. They are QR codes (Quick Response) and by scanning them with your smartphone, you can see more stuff. They will take you to various, safe webpages that augment my thoughts, mostly. Some are just silly. Okay, a lot of them are just silly. Ignore them or scan them with your phones. It's what we like to call in the business "added value." If your phone or tablet doesn't have a QR reader, you can get one for free in the app store or wherever you found *Angry Birds*. Don't worry though, you're not supposed to see patterns in amongst the squares and squiggles. (If you do, maybe consult a doctor or an exorcist.)

Go ahead, give it a try. You can practice on this one. Maybe even leave a note saying hi!
—Rodney

# Dedication:

For my mother who curled up at my bedside (just like she did 47 years ago).

*  *  *

For my Big Brother Dean who gave me the hug of life on that horrible night at Lake Michigan.

*  *  *

For my Big Brother Scott who gave me his stem cells and a plastic army man.

*  *  *

And, as always, for The Lady Macraes.

"Rodney has a magical way of telling the god-awful honest truth in a way that makes readers feel as if, well, life's like that and you might as well enjoy the adventure."

—*Susan Ager, retired columnist, Detroit Free Press*

"Just spent 30 hilarious minutes in the @MichiganRadio studio with @rcurtis #ILoveRadio"

—*Meg Cramer, Public Insight analyst, American Public Media*

CHAPTER **1**

*I wrote the following entry for a blog I was maintaining at the time and waited to publish it until all my test results were done. I was sure all would be fine. I never ended up posting it. That sounds more dire than it really is. If you haven't already guessed, I'm not writing this retrospective from beyond the grave. But hopefully that doesn't dissuade you from reading this. I lived; be happy for me, for crying out loud. What are you, some kind of ghoul?*

# Bone Tired

THE KINDLY DOCTOR was chatting me up about the latest thing he saw on YouTube as he dug around inside my bones looking for some good marrow to harvest. It was more painful hearing about the nicotine-addicted toddler in China than it was getting the tool twisted into my bone and the marrow extracted.

All this because my blood is a little screwed up. When they yanked my gall bladder, a routine blood test showed a low white blood cell count. Subsequent tests showed my red blood cells and hemoglobin were also too low. Great. Excellent. Unemployment, the Gulf oil spill, now this.

No one thinks this is leukemia or lymphoma. My first doctor actually laughed at me when I mentioned those dreaded words. But the fact remains, the next doctor she sent me to runs The Cancer and Leukemia Center. Looking him up on Google didn't help my fears much when after his name I saw the words "Hospice Care."

So, more tests, more pokes, more prodding and the dude who runs the hospice center said he's 90% sure my "illness" is just due to me being Rodney. "That's just the way your body works; sometimes it's up, sometimes it's down," he said.

But he prescribed the bone marrow test.

Lying there on the gurney with my butt exposed to the German technician, the Asian hematologist and the nurse from Troy, I realized I was truly having a worldly experience. Talking about the dopey things on YouTube was our common language. Fear of Cancer was on another channel.

He—the doctor jabbing things into my hip—also scoffed at this being serious. "Look, if you don't have enlarged organs and aren't feeling weird in any part of your body, this is probably just a cyclical thing that normally happens with you."

He went on to explain that like unemployment and other forces, this too was just part of a natural ebb and flow. I liked that. Yeah, I groove on Eastern philosophy, especially when it's being quoted by an Eastern doc who's digging around inside of me like a prospector staking his claim.

So why worry about bad, horrible results when three doctors now assure me it's nothing?

I think it's because they don't give blood tests and bone marrow extractions to random passersby on the street. You have to earn the privilege.

Actually, if the doctors' assurances didn't allay my fears, a psychic's palm reading helped. She had a sandwich board outside her parlor advertising $15 readings. She said my life line is long and strong so phew, I'm good. She also said I love traveling, have a huge load of money rushing my way and that, strangely, I enjoy slow cookers.

Stop Rodney, stop. The slow cooking thing is a lie. But it was a fun diversion and I take every opportunity these days to distract myself.

It's easy during the day to rationalize my condition into nothing more than a mere oddity. I pound it with everything I have, including white light, God, favors from deceased family and friends and yes, that nutty psychic who also told me a personal truth that no one else knows.

But in the mysterious dark of night, when strange dreams of Montel Williams shake me awake, the thing I fear most is not death, but leaving my daughters stranded. Being as honest as humanly possible, that fear is the one I can't live with. My mom's mom died when my mother and her twin were 15. My daughters, Taylor and Skye, are 14 and 16 now. The only way I'm abandoning this journey is if my daughters get all Lyle and Erik Menendez (*http://bit.ly/102TECK*) on me.

Otherwise, leukemia, lymphoma or even a lobotomy stand no chance against me, the psychic and every doctor so far who's laughed at my fears.

CHAPTER 2

# The L-Word

WHEN LIFE IS totally uncool, make Kool-Aid.
Why lead with humor? Just jump right in with the facts; I have leukemia.
There you go; that wasn't so difficult, was it? Okay, the hard part's over. Plow through. When I was having my gall bladder yanked out recently, one of the blood tests came back with a creepy sounding phrase, "your white blood cell count is low."
Ever since the operation, subsequent tests have shown it dropping even lower. I can't help thinking about that Flo Rida (*http://bit.ly/SbcO6c*) song. Low, low, low, low …
Great, you're quoting pop culture from a few years ago. That's the Rodney we know and love.
No one thought I could have leukemia, particularly since I'm showing no signs of it whatsoever. Every single question the doctors have asked has been met with an easy "nope." One guy even glanced nervously at my wife, Marci, when he wondered aloud about HIV.
"Nope."

But here it sits inside my body. Acute Myeloid Leukemia.

I'm told the cure rate is very high and if I simply *must* have leukemia, this is the one to have. I like the fact that it's acute. A cutie. Awww, look how cute that leukemia is, don't you just wanna reach out and, and, smash it with a sledge hammer?

I'm in the hospital and have checked in for about a month. Whoa, a month? Did I really just write that? Summer. Cherries. Daughters out of school. Camping. Leukemia.

It sounds like Bohemia. It sounds like bulimia. It sounds like I'll be doing a lot of that as they pump poison into my body and I throw up. Ewww, and then my hair.

I have a few aces in the hole though. This is highly treatable and the remission rates are in my favor. Being very healthy going into this makes it easier, supposedly. My doctor has seen more cancer patients than anyone in the area, he claims, and he stared me in the eyes while saying I was going to be fine and get better. Maybe better than I ever was before. I'll be Steve Austin (the Bionic Man, not the wrestler).

I have another ace and I called her on the Batphone. You only call her when you really need her. She is the director of blood and marrow at The Mayo Clinic and she is my kindly Aunt Roberta. "It's not going to be a walk in the park," she told me. "But keep feeling like Rodney; try not to feel like a patient." Those are great words. I'd rather feel like Rodney. So I've been making jokes about it, including on the video I made for my daughters where I said, "Let's lick leukemia," then quickly retracted it because, ugh, that just sounds disgusting.

I ordered an iPad, which made my wife instantly suspicious of this whole leukemia ruse. When the doctor said he also loved Cappuccino Blasts and I could drink them with reckless abandon, Marci knew the fix was in.

Friends and family have begun offering prayers and wonderful sentiments. So far, though, the people that need the prayers more are the bottom third of the Tiger's lineup. I'm fine. I'm going to destroy this dis-ease. The bottom of the

chapter 2 • 5

Tiger's batting order? I honestly don't know about their prognosis.

I'll find a better phrase than "Let's lick leukemia," but in the meantime my working phrase is "I have a 'cute' leukemia." Nothing makes cancer madder than belittling it and pinching its darling baby cheeks.

CHAPTER 3

# Having Fun with Cancer

THE HEAD NURSE walked into my room and did one of those classic sitcom double takes. "What the ..." she said as she scanned my visitors.

"Are all of you sick?" She looked over at me, smiling in the chair, with my trusty pole-dance partner Ivy standing next to me, pumping her poison gently into my veins.

"He's the one that's supposed to be wearing the mask, not all of you," she said, pointing to me.

"Oh, Rodney..." and you could almost hear the *wuh waaah* of the soundtrack and the audience laughing (*http://bit.ly/UNckkK*) as my guests realized they'd been duped. Then I busted out my own personalized hygienic mask with a giant smile and two gapped teeth drawn in the middle with a Sharpie.

My brother got me back though. He's seven years older and has always gotten me back. When the sweet Ukrainian nurse came in to take my blood, she said thickly and kindly, "I use small needle. You poked too many times."

My brother Scott said, "No, it's okay, he likes the bigger needles." Then, as if she were in on the joke he continued, "Rodney, why doesn't she use the kind you normally use for heroin?"

Very soon thereafter, my mother showed up and it was as if we were in the backseat of her car in the 1970s. "Boys, that is **not** funny."

I'll tell you what *is* funny. When I woke up to pee for the 19th time, I decided to commit this previous memory to pixelated paper. I Googled "what is the sound in sitcoms when Gilligan does something dumb." When I clicked on the responses, other things popped up. They weren't pornography, but they were definitely gateways to pornography. Just then, the night nurse burst into my room and you wouldn't believe how quickly a guy with a supposedly life-threatening disease could close windows and make his screen look innocuous.

Some of the people on this ward get my humor instantly. Even the nurse who had cancer herself 25 years ago likes my style. She pulled me aside and said, "I knew instantly you, too, were a survivor. You've already got this thing beat."

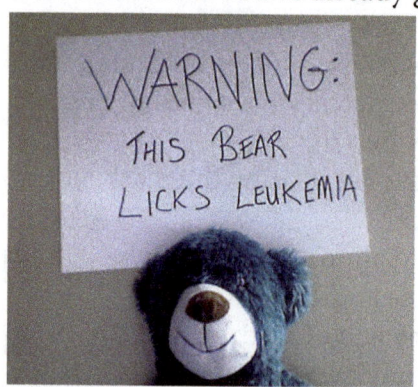

**My daughter's bear sits next to my bed performing his mission.**

But I need to watch my idioms, metaphors and cultural references with some of the foreign staff members. I also need to just plain shut up sometimes. As I was being prepped for surgery this afternoon, to install a port to make it easier for them to poison me, they checked my chart and said, "Oh, you're allergic to shellfish."

That was all due to a flippant comment I made back when I had my gall bladder taken out at this same hospital. I think they asked if had any allergies and I said I didn't want a SpongeBob Band-Aid since I'm allergic to seafood.

That snapped me back to reality. The next question was about having a latex allergy. I bit my tongue when I really, really wanted to answer, "No, but I do have a latex fetish."

To that end, I probably shouldn't make any comment about the conversation I had with the nurse's desk this morning about showering. It went something like this:

"Should you unplug me or cover up the tubes going into my chest while I shower?" I asked.

"Yes, definitely. We wouldn't want anything to leak out of your tubes. That stuff's dangerous; you don't want any of it getting on you. That could be really bad."

The fact that I'm imbibing it intravenously by the quart seemed lost on them.

Something must be working though. My attitude must be having an effect, because that blood taken by the Ukrainian nurse indicated a slight increase in my white cells. That hasn't happened at all during the past six weeks of free-fall. Sure, they're obliterating them as they carpet-bomb my system, but that one little victory gave me a kind of boost I just can't describe.

CHAPTER 4

# Blue Evening

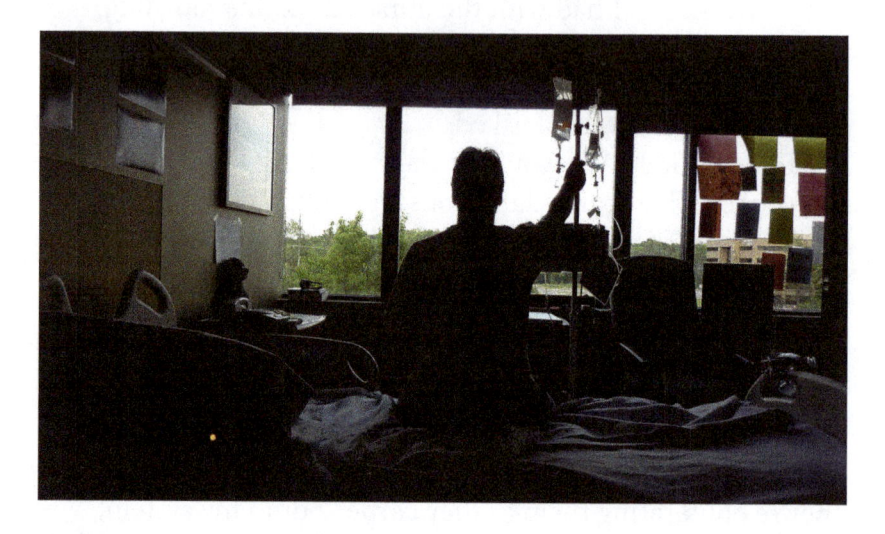

DRIP … DRIP … drip … go the toxic chemicals that are killing all my bone marrow cells, good and bad. And as I lay here feeling physically fine, I miss my boring ordinary Sunday night family routine. Marci's editing pictures, Skye is taking a shower, Taylor is working on some last bits of homework and I yearn to be part of the subtle sway of my home filled with females.

My doctor, a wonderful man from India, knows in his gut that he'll have good news for me about my bone marrow on Tuesday, "But I want to see it on paper in front of me." I too can visualize him reporting, with a smile, that they caught this infiltration early enough so a total and complete cure is in sight.

The incredible support I've received from family and long-time friends, as well as brand new folks who have just appeared in my life, is staggering. You don't always know how truly connected you are until an event like this transpires and suddenly you are invited to see a rare glimpse of how humanity actually works. My wife wrote on her Facebook wall that she didn't realize all 479 of my "friends" were actually friends without the quotation marks. It has made my blue, sad, tearful jags briefer and almost silly in a way. How can I get down when everyone is rallying around me?

There have been acts of amazing kindness, extreme silliness, and just plain sweetness. Tonight our friends, the Radkes, brought me a basket of suckers with the phrase **"Let's Lick Leukemia"** stuck onto every stick.

In my funkiest of funks I wonder why this is happening: did I really just have nothing else to do, was I *that* in need of new things to write about, or did I piss off the devil with that 666 story I wrote in my previous book?

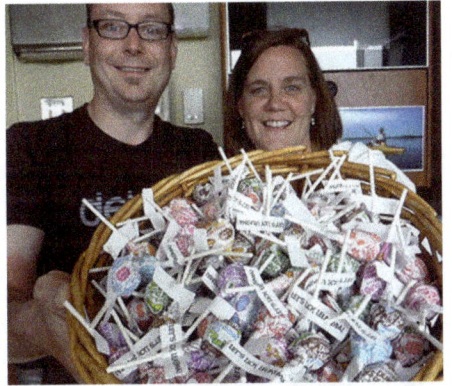

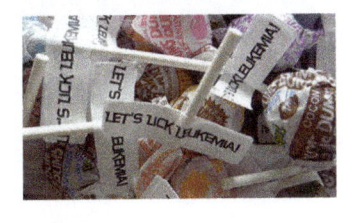

But then the eternal optimist in me grabs hold of my hair (the hair that I'm told will soon be vacating the premises) and says, "Look, Bud, it's because you had nothing else going on that you cleared the time to listen to your body and caught this early on."

The guy down the hall from me has been in and out since January because he showed up in emergency back then with pneumonia. He has exactly what I have. His hair grew back, then he lost it again because he caught another infection and was back here for another round and on and on. But the thing

chapter 4 • 11

is, he's fine. He's much older than I am and yes, I'm taking comfort in other people's stories.

I'm rambling. I can tell. I've seen this in me before so I'll pull these horses to a halt and circle the wagons for the night. I'll take one more self portrait to give you the mood I'm feeling tonight then I'll gratefully accept my first sleeping pill and drift off.

Tuesday can't come soon enough.

CHAPTER 5

# Departure Terminal

THE PARKING LOT is mostly empty at our departure terminal, but the sun still hasn't risen and activity is on hold for now. Most of the shift workers have completed their important duties and are just in monitoring mode, flipping through magazines, making final notes in their endless computer ledgers, waiting.

I and the other "Acute Leuks," as our doctor has named us, have an unofficial handoff too. I don't know exactly what it is but I think we're the watchers.

The Czech gentleman down the hall—who is done with chemo, yet has to stay here due to risk of infection—wanders around the ward in the evening, keeping the nurses awake. I switch off with him during the day and joke around, hand out lollipops and relish the smiles as the care workers—amazingly gifted in their field—walk fast with an unhurried rush to their next call.

We are watching the exiting. We are in some indescribable way here to witness the transformation.

If you walk 17 times around this cancer ward, almost a perfect square in shape, you have completed a mile and the nurses smile and say, "Hey, you didn't let your mom beat you today." But exercise is only a sham. Sure, I want to keep up my muscle mass. But my circuits around the track, while I still have energy, are also done for a deeper reason. I'm looking into the souls of those on the loading platforms and wondering what they're wondering.

Yesterday, a woman my age was clutching her cell phone but not making any calls as she huddled in the darkest corner of turn three. The first time by, I mentioned something light and she responded that her mother just passed on. The second time I slowed and offered her a hug which she seemed to melt into. The third time around, her brother exited the room and they slowly walked away. The fourth time came the "Get Well" balloons, a bit deflated, sure, but still remarkably mylared.

Then she came out.

I slowed. My pace didn't need to be so quick. She was a young woman of 80-something and there she lay on her bed, head cocked to one side, mouth agape, eyes closed and pointing toward her next destination. I didn't feel like a gawker or a ghoul. More like a bon voyage party of one.

Don't get me wrong, I wasn't throwing streamers or striking up celestial bands. But I did get another one of those feelings that tell me deep truths. Her time here was over but this was only one segment of her journey. I don't say this, sitting backwards on my bed, tapping in the pre-dawn light because I want to believe it or wish I thought it. I tell you this because I can actually see it.

That's partly why I'm here. I'm the one that's haunting this place, not them. I'm the one who doesn't belong, but since

I'm being offered this rare glimpse along with the other Acute Leuks I think it's my duty to report back to you as objectively as my subjective mind can.

The bustle of this place will start to hustle. I'll fall back asleep and forget for a moment or two that I woke to write this. I'll try to find something funny to INSERT HERE as I re-read this, just so I can feel more like myself. Don't let me get away with too much though. Don't let me hide too deeply in that Mr. Funny Man persona.

I'm staying back here on the docks and will continue to take my notes. I'm not joining their journeys for a long time yet. Am I glad I get to get a glimpse? *Heavens yes.* Are my bags properly packed for the voyage?

**Hell no.**

CHAPTER **6**

# No News is Good News

"Did you use a Sharpie to make that smiley face? You shouldn't be breathing those fumes," said our family friend Tony as we wandered around the cancer ward.

"What's it gonna do, Tony, gimme cancer?"

And with that, we're back.

All yesterday we were waiting to hear how my little bits of bone marrow were growing. They were popped out of my hip with a corkscrew contraption that Napa Valley would've been proud of and set in a glass dish to multiply, divide, conquer or just party. I've never known what goes on in petri dishes except for those awful science fiction movies where you see little Zac Efron heads grafted onto Selena Gomez bodies. But maybe that was just a YouTube video of their latest date I just saw. The chemo has me a bit befuddled sometimes.

It turns out my marrow is just taking a little while longer to grow and become mature. Cough, cough, gasp? Mature? *My marrow, immature?* No way.

My mother, who is sitting at home with a portable phone in her lap watching Obama's oil spill report, and my wife at her computer were both shocked to hear that we'd have to wait even longer. We'd been waiting all day as it was. So I made sure to use their anxiety as a cover for my own when the doctor strode into my room.

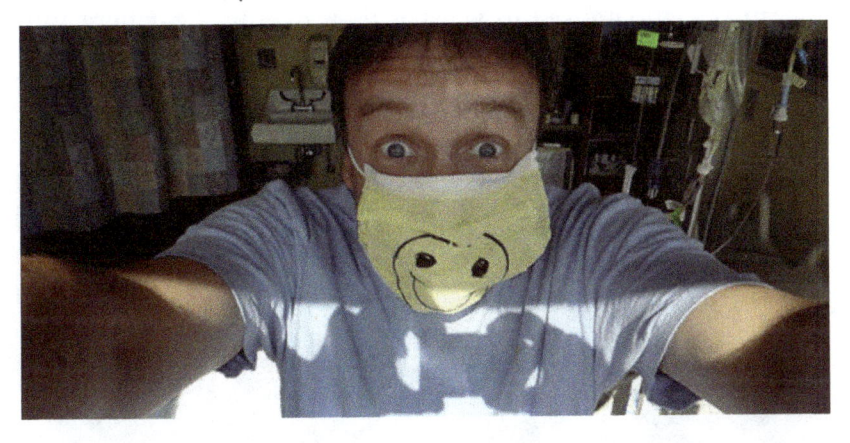

"Look, I tell you again and again, you are fine. Didn't you meet another man today who had this far, far worse than you?" he reminded me.

"Yes, doctor, and he's helped my wife and I find tons of resources already."

"Resources. You don't need resources. You just need to sit here, get bored and get cured." I think I offended him. And like in those old commercials I hoped he wouldn't pull one of those, "It's not nice to offend Mother Nature." (Just go with me on this one, I know it's *fool* Mother Nature, but you get the drift).

I explained that we were just exploring all monetary avenues to help pay for stuff our co-pays and COBRAS and cohorts can't cover and that seemed to assuage him. But the takeaway I got from him, loudly and clearly was, "Hey, this will take a while, but you'll be better."

We're pinning our hopes on how early they caught the disease, even if I have to search for bone marrow, or even if I won't be through this until fall, winter … none of that matters. Right now they are hitting me with hard doses of chemo, because I am healthy and active. Therefore my cell count is lower than the Greek treasury and so my risk of disease just shot through the roof.

"Look at this as a season," said another one of the incredible nurses who chose this ward as their calling. "Stay here and relax. It'll be over soon enough."

Maybe I need to sink into this as a gift and spend time getting in touch with me.

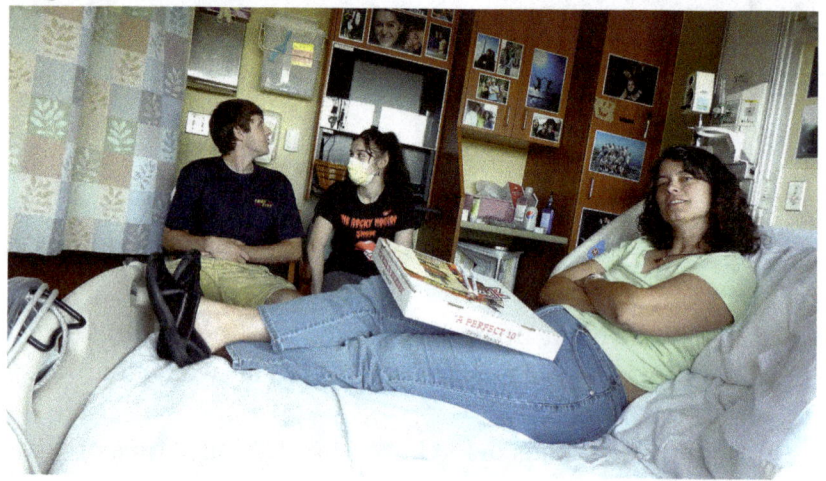

*Eating a bunch of deep, rich, thick, gooey pizza wasn't exactly what the doctor ordered. But then again, he wasn't exactly on the ward when it was delivered by my family. I would've offered him a slice.*

Well, me and my family anyway. Yesterday a fantastic Pizzapapalis (*http://pizzapapalis.com/*) dinner, along with all our teen hangers-on, arrived and we ate like kings right here in this hospital room. Jon, another of our solid family friends, even took it upon himself to scarf down my normal hospital dinner so the nutritional staff wouldn't feel sad. They all played with the iPad, we related wonderful stories about how Taylor was asked to the 8th grade dance, we saw Marci's Google ranking jump up precipitously after a butt-load of work and for a moment or 10 it was just like we were back home, in our kitchen.

Except there were no dogs. And that wasn't necessarily a bad thing.

The results will come. We'll deal with them and move forward. I am sitting here after another great night's sleep (brought on courtesy of a slight injection of Adavan, Aveeda or Avatar for sleeping). And I am awaiting my daily Cappuccino Blast (*http://on.fb.me/Us6LuO*) from Marci who will sneak one in for another day or two until I can't stand the sight of food.

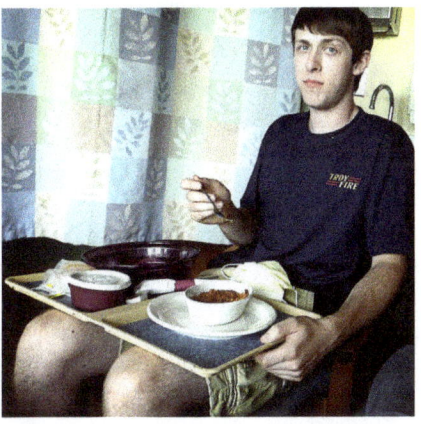

And all is well. Remarkably and totally illogically, I am fine.

CHAPTER **7**

# A Better Medicine

**IT MIGHT NOT** be the healthiest reaction I've had lately, but when I woke up just now, at 4:00 a.m., I felt a giant laugh in my gut. I won't try and kid you that it was an all fun-and-games guffaw; most of you have seen through that charade by now.

It felt more like, *I got laid off exactly a year ago, tried another newspaper which lasted five minutes, found a great teaching gig with amazing students but school cutbacks are coming, our van got totaled and now this—a disease that's cleaning my clock.*

Happy anniversary baby, where do I send the flowers for a fabulous year of living on the edge? There's a pity parade forming along both sides of the street and I think I'm supposed to be the Grand Marshal.

And yet, here's the weirdest fact of all. My odd doctor pushed into the room without knocking and said two simple words, "normal cytogenetics." Not being able to comprehend what that meant, I had to collar him for more information.

"Your leukemia is *de novo*, which means it just came from out of the blue. This is not a bad prognosis," he said in his wonderful Indian voice.

There is something inside me though, maybe brought on by the past year's turmoil but most likely just a general *Rodney thing* that's doing battle with this supposedly good news. When he said, "this is not a bad prognosis," did he really mean it could be worse? When he said the risk of the disease returning was intermediate, did he mean if we only napalmed the village once? Or should I just hold tight to the last image of him walking away from me with both hands pumped into the air like a World Cup midfielder?

Everything is good so far. I have 46 XY chromosomes and right now, the ones in my bones are being blasted long and hard by bag after bag of a poison so toxic, I have to actually flush the toilet twice each time I pee to push the chemicals further down deep into the Beaumont Hospital sewers. Seriously.

Thankfully, this first round of chemo*scarepy* is coming to an end tomorrow.

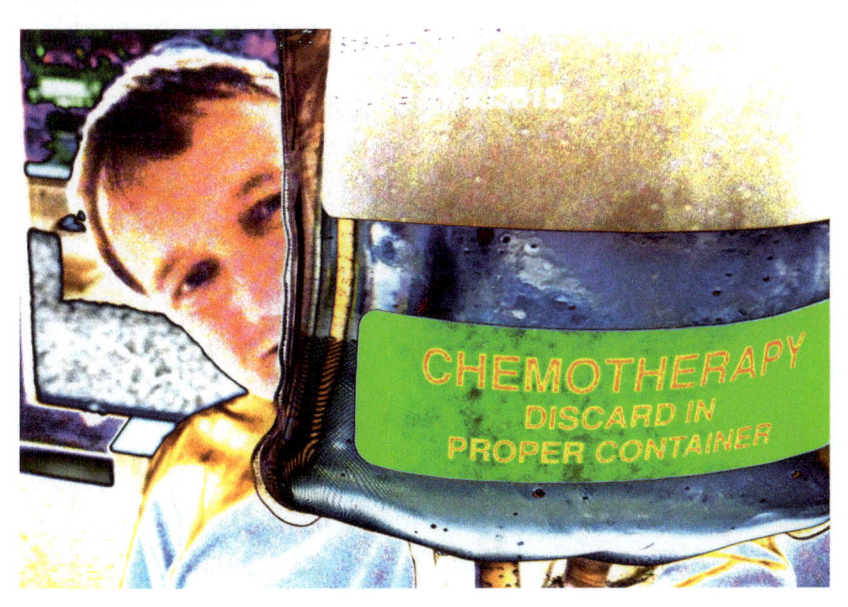

I wish that analogy got to the heart of my malaise. I wish, too I could blame this latest funk because I'm drunk on junk.

My wife said, "You really wanted this all to be just a big mistake and be told it was only mono."

Yeah. That's part of it. But I guess there's the whole victim element that plays into this too. God knows I've always loved being the center of attention. But equally so, I've always wanted to control the story, to say it in my own way. I've never wanted to let the news dictate me and unfortunately it's starting to … or I feel it's starting to. Taking control over my rotten layoff this past year has given me a little voice in my own destination. Writing about this ludicrous leukemia can hopefully do the same.

So I'm folding up the chairs and putting the streamers for the pity parade back into storage. Hell, I may even flush them into the hospital sewer. Yes, I had hoped this would be over and done with by mid-summer and I could celebrate with a nice Dragonmead Trippel Ale (*http://www.dragonmead.com/*). It's ironic, yet highly appropriate, that my favorite brand, the kind I crave more than any other draft from their microbrewery lineup is called Final Absolution.

The deep laughter starts rolling again. And trust me, this time it's real.

CHAPTER 8

# Chemo Sabes

I MAY BE crashing soon. Chemo's last stage is willfully pumping its final, fatal fluid into my bones and even though I'm still walking my mile laps around the ward, my feet have gotten sloggy, as if for lack of another place to go, the liquid has opted to kill my stride as well.

Cancer survivors tell me to not feel obligated to *anything* or *anyone* but me. I hear over and over again that once this first round drags every muscle fragment and creative impulse into a deep, dark abyss I won't want to be jolly blogging about SpongeBob or jokes I played on my brother. I understand that in my head.

But the other side of that scenario is my extreme need for connection and my almost psychotic need to interact and share. I looked up "sociopath" to see if it has an opposite and there really isn't one. Might as well insert my picture there, then.

I was just told that in the old building where I used to work—in the lobby between the *Detroit Free Press* and *Detroit*

*News*—there's a dry erase idea board that says to send good vibes my way. I thought I'd used up all my happy tears days ago.

Another part of this connection equation is my Aunt Roberta, with whom I shared the bone marrow report. Suddenly I was a young teen boy again, looking up to my amazing, powerful aunt as I wrote:

*"I was gladdened by the results, hopefully not blindly. Everything is good so far; does that sound hopeful? Please say yes."*

With a large exclamation point she wrote back, "Yes!"

She was just jumping on a plane and will have more information for me later but it shows how we thrive on the people bouncing through our lives for a day or a decade. It had been a year since I had any long-term, sit-down conversation with Roberta and yet with a few simple words I am carried to a place that's impossible to go alone.

And while we're at it, that dry erase board in the newspaper lobby marks, I'm certain, one of the last sites I saw as I was gently told to leave a year ago due to layoff. Now people are using it to send me positive energy. That is an absolutely astounding mandate on the power of connectivity.

Here's just as a little parable to end this: Think of what can happen when you believe you're connected to something but really and truly aren't. I wish I knew ahead of time that I was in a part cancer/part hospice ward. I think it would've explained all the deaths going on around me in a more natural way and I wouldn't have been so freaked out by the low success rates here if I knew *success* was being measured in how comfortable the patient's final stay was and how incredible the nurses were.

Maybe they told me earlier. Maybe I was in no place to listen. I'm not going anywhere for a long time but it was beginning to get me down until I just simply asked.

So take it from the cancer boy in Room 2603. This journey is about the people you collect along the way. I'll see what more I can write and when I can write it. Heck, the sunrise was beautiful for the first time all week and since it just happens to signify the end of round one, I'll tip my ice-water glass to all of you. Thank you for wandering with me during this initial round of chemotherapy. I couldn't have done it without you.

These boots are made of cancer, and I'm just gonna slog through.

CHAPTER **9**

# Five Laps

**F**IVE LAPS AROUND the cancer ward.
Five laps takes you past the little girl with eyes too big to see Grandma slyly slipping away.
Five laps will exercise your bones just enough to let the chemotherapy keep destroying you.
Five laps and you can't go on because next door, right next door, an old man is talking loudly on his cellphone to his brother about their sister's last moments.
If you don't do your laps, you stay in your room and forget.
When you do your laps you see your normal nurses but you see the other ones too. They speak in foreign tongues, hushing into rooms.
Five laps around the cancer ward where people with eyes wider than yours on your first day stare out silently asking "What the **HELL?!**"
Laptops are plugged in everywhere as if somehow a video conference with eternity will be interrupted by a governor's pardon.

I don't know if people can see me.

I don't know if I exist as I spook their halls.

Five miles away is ice cream and movies and daughters and, and, and ...

Five laps down. Five million more.

CHAPTER **10**

# Dear Nephew

YOU ARE THE youngest, newest member of our vast, crazy family and your great-uncle Rodney has a funny story to tell. Well, by the end of this you may not think of me as "great" per say; everyone just calls me Uncle Rodney anyway, even if they're my cousins or not technically even related to me.

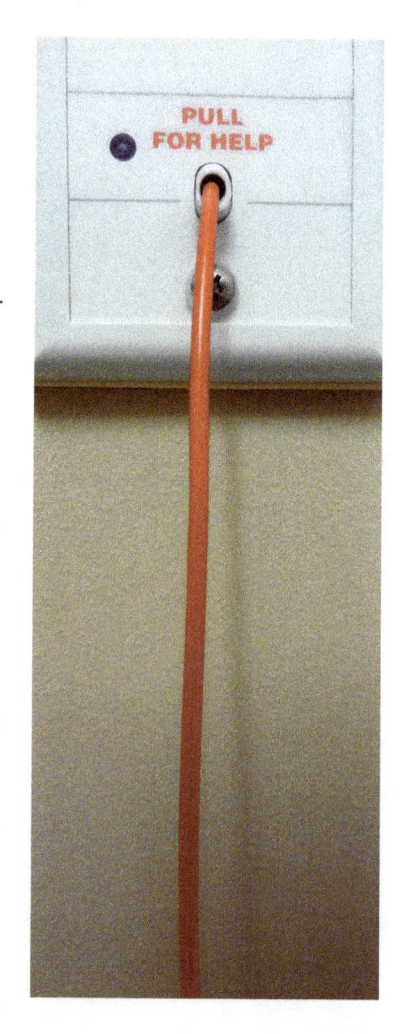

I am in the hospital right now with a disease that finds new and highly creative ways each night to kick my butt. Oops, you're not even a one-year-old yet; I shouldn't curse. This disease is beating me up. But in the end I am going to win, so the story already has a happy ending.

So Colin, you're probably still in diapers now, right? The wonderful thing about diapers is you can play, play, play all day and when you need to go potty, you just do. Take my advice, my nephew, stay in diapers as long as possible. No, I'm not writing to tell you Uncle Rodney is in diapers, that would be silly. I'm writing to say how I fainted on the potty last night.

You've seen potties; Mommy and Daddy have a few of them and they seem so big and bright and white and make noise at the end. Well Colin dear, it's completely understandable—to me anyway—if you'd like to wait on what they call "toilet training." I thought I was toilet trained until last night at 2:00 a.m. when the whole hospital code staff, emergency room workers and everyone on my floor was crowded into my room because I lost consciousness while pooing.

Hospitals have emergency cords right next to the toilets. I can't describe, Colin, exactly how I knew to pull the cord. But when my head was snapping back and forth and I couldn't focus, apparently I knew I had to pull the ripcord.

There are some wonderful people on this planet. Many of them were in my room last night. I kept hearing my name over and over again until finally I just opened my eyes and looked out to see them all. Somehow they had gotten me to my bed, attached machines all over me and even had those crazy **"Clear"** paddles you may have seen on one of Mom's scary nighttime shows.

I was fine. They gave me all sorts of good things to make me better and last night was just a funny memory.

And really Colin, that's why I'm writing. I know you're too young to interpret this and I'm just using a cheap literary device to tell a story, but it's my story. I can laugh if I want to. So many people today have said, "you must've been so scared."

But I wasn't and I'm not.

And that's the thing about growing up in this family. You will be told things all the time about how to be and how to react, but, little dude, you get to make up your own rules as you go along. You will feel how you feel for no other reason than *that's the way you feel.*

I think too, there's something else lurking in my mind. Let me try and pin it down. Treatment for the disease I have has progressed so far in recent years. Right now, the very best of our medicine says to kill all the junk in my bones and let my body grow back the good stuff. I bet ... I *know* that by the time you've grown up they'll figure out a way to just destroy the bad stuff in people and leave the good things safe and secure. But more importantly, let's hope for a time where this disease never even starts.

Write your own story, my wonderful nephew. Write it every day with surprises and fun. But know there may be times when you need to pull the ripcord. And when you do, there will be so many of us rushing in to help, it will make your head spin with love.

# CHAPTER 11

# Ode to an Egg Salad Sandwich

I LOOK AT you there, decimated, crusts hanging akimbo. My first solid meal in three days. You were a hero to me and I returned the favor by savagely tearing you apart in a way most maniacal.

Like classic theatrical masks, half of you smiles at me, the other frowns. Comedy within the tragedy.

While your life ends, you bring new hope and life to my digestive tract, ravaged by fluids so vile we daren't speak their name. Soft ice cream preceded you, mayhaps Pei Wei will follow.

Ahh, but I cheapen your departure with disrespect. Your taste lingers. Your effect courses through me. The power of your simple concoction thrills me like no sandwich has ever before.

Know this sir, know this as surely as you course through me; you were a friend. And I bow to you even now as your crust and crumbs become one inside me.

Contentment spreads from your essence. Happiness flows from you. Energy, strength and a true willingness to continue are your legacy.

CHAPTER **12**

# Half a Dozen Cupcakes

THE DAY DIDN'T start out well for me. There was an unusual amount of hair that had decided today was the day to end it all on the dry salt flats of my pillow. And the pounding headaches of the night before were telling me the poison was doing its work in the swanky penthouse upstairs where my brain entertains dignitaries, holds court with Bono and Sting, taps out bestsellers and does things I'll keep to myself, thank you very much.

The last thing I wanted was visitors.

Or cupcakes.

And after my mom, my niece and my wife came by, my hospital bed called to me. That's exactly when dear friend Patty Montemurri showed up at my room with six designer cupcakes. You have to understand, newsrooms and baked goods go together like Woodward and Bernstein (or Elrick and Schaefer (*http://on.freep.com/TV34Kl*)).

I'm sick. It's not the leukemia though, it's now the lack of an immune system. Don't get me wrong, it doesn't feel like the flu or a cold, but if you bring in a stray spore from New Baltimore, it can turn into pneumonia. Not to put too fine a point on it, I have no grime-fighting ability; neither bleach nor borax.

Patty and I chatted, of course. She's too wonderful a person to blow off. We became buddies at "that newspaper that laid me off." She told me about the nuns who have me on their prayer wall and that no more layoffs were coming in the near future.

We oohed and ahhed over the cupcakes but she kept changing the place of the secondary thing, a large envelope in the shape of, yes, a cupcake as well.

*Get that filthy thing off my bed*, I kept thinking. *Do you have any idea where that could've been?* sounding like parents the world over.

It was obvious the gaudy cupcake was more important than our conversation so I reluctantly pulled on some rubber gloves and had a look.

*Great, a card. How nice,* I snidely continued in my head. The last time I got cards and baked goods from the *Free Press* was a year ago this week as I was shown the door. But the warmth in their greeting card messages then was sweeter and more potent to my soul than the delicious parties thrown for me by two entirely different departments.

Okay, sure, I'll play the game we all play with Hallmark. You look at the cutesy message on the front and try to figure out what the punch line will be. I didn't do so well.

I, the purveyor of punch lines, was punched right back with a sucker blow so unseen, so un-telegraphed that now, hours later, I'm astounded at its power. It pushed a year's worth of anger at my former corporation out into the cancer ward and down into the sewers festering with expelled chemo.

34 • A "Cute" Leukemia

Spilling from the card, along with the extra pages added due to too many greetings, were an insane number of portraits of pursed-lipped statesman Ben Franklin. And they were rectangular. And they were green.

"It's from everyone," Patty said, "from those who actually laid you off, to people who just care."

Here's where I'll pause for a brief note to all the guys out there. If you haven't expelled tears or feel weird crying, you really need to give it a shot, and soon. Yes, you'll probably do it alone, hidden in some deep corner of thought because that's the way real men do things. But cry, dammit. Let it out; you'll feel the positive effect within 10 seconds.

Convulsive waves washed over me and after time stopped standing still, I went in for the hug. A masked, horrified Patty recoiled due to my litany about germs, but there was something cosmically antiseptic in the air right then and I wasn't going to be denied.

Here's where I'll pause one last time to say a cheap, far-too-cliché thank you to everyone at my former place of work. I don't know if you realize it or not, but that family you're part of—that family that we're part of—sticks with you in ways both profound and pastry.

OK, I'm looking for a way that Benjamin Franklin can wrap this up, but I can't seem to manipulate any of his quotes to do my bidding. Maybe he'll come through later, like a stitch in time.

Newspapers are not corporations; they are made from the talent and excitement of individual people. It took me too much time to remember that. Every newsroom I've ever worked for has shared surprising and fun moments with me. Oh, and the readers, too.

Journalists are going through some intensive soul-searching. Everyone's trying to figure out how to save the industry. With the amazing spirit that so many of my sisters and brothers possess, here's to hoping somebody will find an answer or a way out of the tailspin.

chapter 12 • 35

Where's Ben Franklin when we really need him? Well for me anyway, he's securely tucked—with his brothers—in the Beaumont Hospital safe.

CHAPTER **13**

# Hair Today, Gone Tomorrow

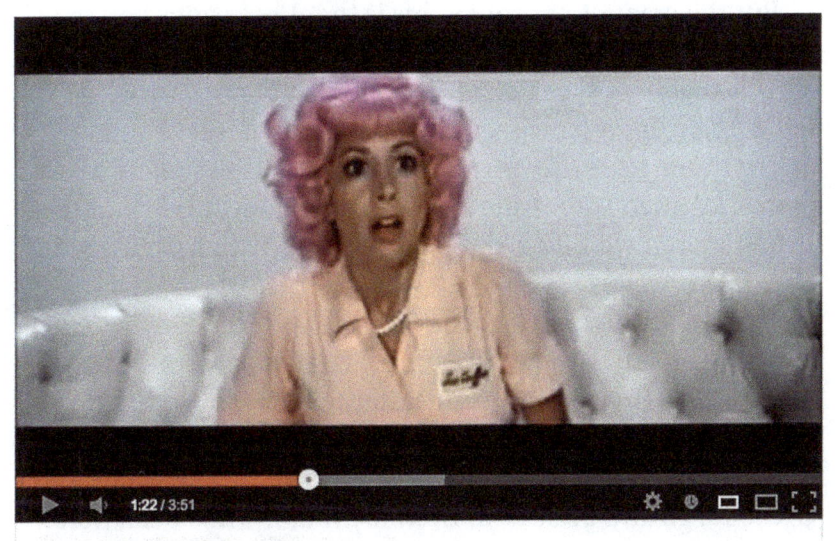

beauty school drop out grease

**HAIR ON YOUR** pillowcase in the morning is one thing. Hair on your keyboard is quite another. That's it, I'm getting a buzz cut.

All along, my daughters have been waiting with itchy clipper fingers to jump in and create fun and strange designs with my hair. They're getting their opportunity this afternoon, with Marci's supervision, to play Beauty School Dropout (*http://bit.ly/Z8YyOJ*), with my head as the victim.

What they deign to leave—which hopefully is just a buzz cut and not that freaky airbender (*http://bit.ly/TV339i*) thing Taylor keeps talking about—will fall out soon enough anyway. I know this now due to some amazingly candid help from cancer-buddy Jan Lovell, with whom I used to work at *The Detroit News*. Jan had a full beard and a thick head of hair into his sixties, which he lost about a year ago, then grew back. He was laid off too. Yeah, we have some commonality.

But the craziest part of all this is that I hear guys have a tougher time, emotionally, with the hair loss than women. How is that possible? Person after person I speak with says female cancer patients seem to have a quiet reserve and are fine with the loss whereas they typically see guys going all to pieces. Women who pride themselves on long, luxurious locks seem to handle it better than guys like me with haircuts left over from the 70s.

It just goes to reinforce one of my long-term core beliefs that women are stronger than men. My ladies are proof positive of this. They have a tremendous power within them to handle this cancer talk without getting too freaked out or worried about the future. And yet, they seem to know when it's OK to let go and be scared. Even my mom, who's been here daily because she can't stand to be anywhere else, openly shares her fears but also her fierce Rodney advocacy.

With all the crap that's been handed our family this year, there have been a lot of equal and opposite reactions to that crap. In that respect, Skye's been going around quoting Sarah Silverman. "When life hands you AIDS, you just gotta make lemonaids."

Sick, yes. Funny, definitely!

CHAPTER **14**

# Bad News/Good (Detroit) News

When you get blindsided, your first reaction always seems to be, "Why didn't I see that coming?" But that's the very definition of being blindsided. That's why it's not called "frontvisioned." Finding out I had to go back to square one with my chemotherapy blindsided me. I knew it was possible; I just wanted the original "induction" chemo to have done more. What happened next did blindside me. But in a good way.

So after last night's results told me I had to re-navigate the treacherous waters in the Tropic of Cancer, I slept lousily, thinking all the worst possible thoughts of my outcome and woke with a fever, then later a migraine. My family didn't sleep well either. Something about hearing you have to start over makes you begin to see this in a new light.

My new light is destroying leukemia. I'm done with silly games and trying to belittle it. They've changed the regimen and the chemistry so as to maximize destruction. Leukemia, you're going down.

As I was forming my attack plan and the nurses were hanging the many bags onto Ivy, good buddy Chris Farina called and wanted to visit. I was golfing with Chris the morning I got my diagnosis and, as I often tell disbelieving people, I felt *that* good beforehand. Everyone I've spoken with who's had this disease all say they were sick when diagnosed. I was highly unusual; go figure.

Seeing Chris made me happy. We'd instantly become friends at *The Detroit News*; our families have vacationed together and he's great to just hang out with. When I abruptly left the *News* for the *Free Press*, by simply walking down two flights of stairs I always felt like I was abandoning my friends at the *News*.

Chris and I spoke about how he assumed I'd look a lot worse, to which I absentmindedly rubbed my hand across my almost blank skull. We talked about both of our fathers dying of cancer and how this leukemia just became a bit more of a force to be reckoned with. But we also talked about movies, newspaper gossip and I showed him how www.detnews.com (*http://www.detroitnews.com/*) looks on my iPad.

Then I got blindsided.

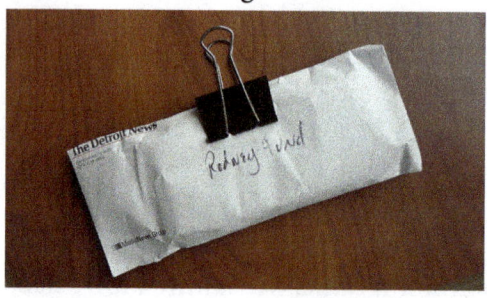

As he was fixing to leave, he leaned to one side and whipped out a Detroit News/Media News Group envelope stuffed with something and held together with a large office paper clamp. It took a moment to comprehend what he was handing me but after two, maybe four seconds, the seismic upheavals began in my gut and erupted out of me as full-on tears. **The News had taken up a collection for me too, just like the Free Press had**.

40 • A "Cute" Leukemia

And they had started it way back before even knowing about each other. The Rodney Fund.

I won't dwell on tears again. They make us feel better and cope easier. But I will say, like the Eskimo words for snow, they break down into many different categories. Today's were along the wonderment vein. My Aunt Roberta sent along a Navajo cure word from back when she worked as a doctor on the reservation. *Chaauh*. I like the way it sounds.

Today, a fellow Michigan Press photographer died of cancer. He admittedly smoked too much and lung cancer did him in. I also learned about another colleague who was just diagnosed with colon cancer. Man, it's not a good run for us shooters. But, as my mom says, within everything we've experienced there's something to be grateful about. John Kaplan, yet another photog with cancer, sent me his amazing video about his battle with the disease. You want to see hope and gratefulness, just check out his story (*http://bit.ly/139v41H*).

But here's my personal note to the entire *Detroit News* staff. First of all, thank you so much for your incredible gift. Expenses are popping up in strange, unforeseen places. My cell phone bill is through the roof but due to the kindness of colleagues, we are able to pay for things like that. Second, I know you all worry about what's next in the journalism business. But take it from me, enjoy the right now and if you have to think about the future, do it in positive ways. Don't ask what you could do to survive, ask what you've really always wanted to do (apart from telling incredible stories). And third, thank you for not resenting me for leaving on that April morning four years ago.

Mostly though, take a look around you at some of the faces you work with every day on the third and fourth floors. Realize that these people are there for you en masse when the chips are down. Even if you can't believe it—even if you walk out on them with no warning—they will shock you with their kindness and outreach and love.

And love.

chapter 14 • 41

CHAPTER **15**

# Maybe a Wasp Took It

THERE'S A FAMOUS story in our family. It's the late 1960s, Yellow Springs, Ohio. My brother Scott and cousin Chris play with plastic army men. Chris's soldier disappears. Scott is blamed. Scott is always blamed. "Maybe a wasp took it," he responds.

Today, a few wasps buzz by my window from an unseen papier-mâché colony. Outside, on the 1st-floor roof, the 2nd-story men walk by, looking for the wasps.

It's a preposterous notion, an insect carrying away a member of the U.S. Armed Forces. No matter how tiny, he's still a Marine. Special Forces, I'm guessing. Whoo-ah.

Outside, the working men walk by, looking at cooling units.

Kids see things as right or wrong, black or white. Secretly, adults do too. Health is right, leukemia is wrong. Crack me open, you'll find health. Leukemia is a game of army men. The tiny, stolen Marine sets fire to my marrow. The disease is like tinder, like kindling, like kerosene flaring up as he patrols my bones, faceless.

Outside, the working men walk by, looking for leaks.

My cousin and brother haven't stopped squabbling about the MIA soldier lost in the Ohio jungles. Both will be tested, though, for marrow matches. Our identical twin mothers make it seem plausible. I'm lucky; I'm Caucasian. Matches aplenty are possible. I'm a WASP. My soul is pained for my brothers and cousins of different races who are so much less likely to find a match.

The little green man, either kneeling or lying down or most likely crouched, carrying a flame thrower, has set a fire circle around my hips and pelvis. There lies the biggest concentration of bone. How the man with no face laughs. He's calling out to the disease, mocking it. "Suck it mutha sucka."

Pardon his French.

Those wasps at the window want to carry him away.

Each rib is a curvy trench. Each toe a foxhole. He's Special Forces; he knows the hiding places. Grenades the size of molded plastic dots are thrown into the dicier areas. Snap, crackle, pop; Cancer Krispies.

Thanks for the soldier, Scott. You knew way back then that your little brother would need him. Sorry Chris, I'll buy you a whole new platoon.

Outside, the working men work.

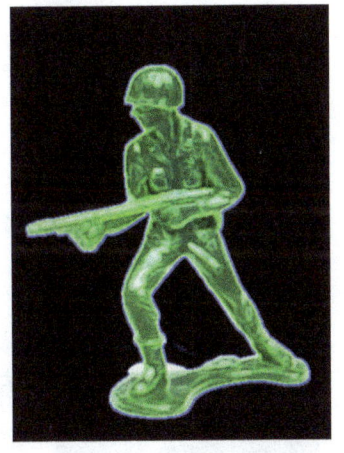

chapter 15 • 43

CHAPTER **16**

# Clown Collage

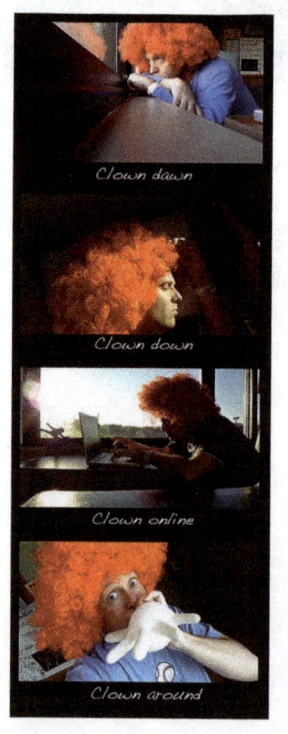

*Clown dawn*

*Clown down*

*Clown online*

*Clown around*

**YESTERDAY MARKED THE** arrival of three incredibly strange gifts. Peter Ross—the buddy I met the same time I met Marci back in '87—sent me an outrageous clown wig from his home in NYC. Long-time pal Kyle Keener created an epic barf bucket with images so inappropriate, I'd better not show you one smidge of its majestic decorations. And Angela Lackey, whom I worked with at the *Midland Daily News*, brought me an okra-colored frog. Incongruous gifts for an incongruous disease.

Wearing the wig out to the nurse's station won me a free outdoor pass for a couple hours. My mom and brother were here (after he entered the room with a crouching army man, presumably **not** the one from the 60s) so they wandered in the glorious holiday weekend sunshine with me.

Do me a favor; at some point lie down on the grass and look up at the fluttery leaves with the sun blue behind them and tell me if they look as silver and magic to you as they did to me.

CHAPTER **17**

# This is ENN

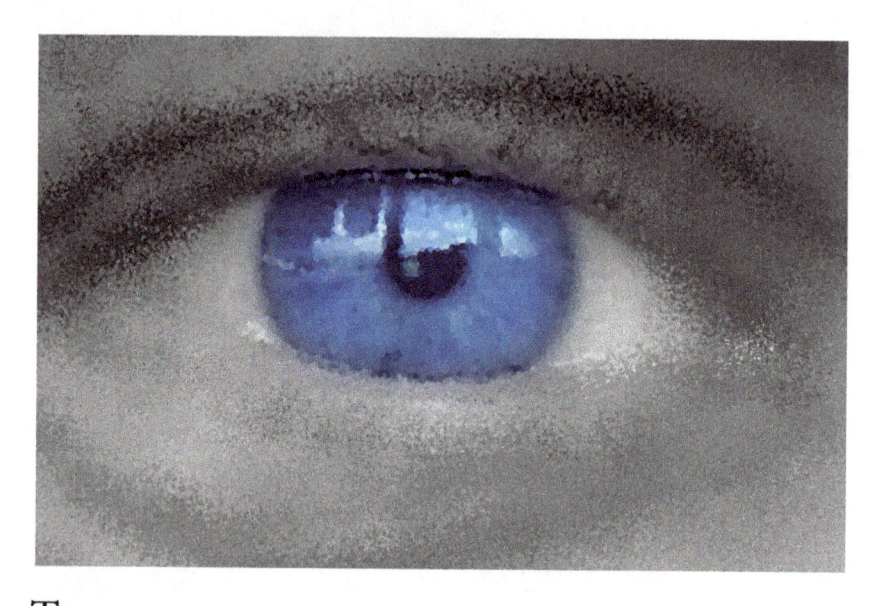

**THEY BURST INTO** my room on stars, trailing unseen comets, the three-person team from "Eternity Network News." Moments earlier I was simply conversing with the great Unknown, explaining why I knew death wasn't near. Our conversation had been delightful and I think I impressed the Unknown. But then these yahoos showed up.

The interviewer sported the latest iPhone 9G, the camera dude recorded it in strict holographic 4-D, but the sound technician was the weirdest; she just used an old microphone from Vaudeville days. They were aggressive, rude and wanted the story. They had deadlines to meet in many different dimensions and even though this happened years or moments ago, they just now sent me the transcripts. I think I did pretty well for being pushed into the spotlight.

**ENN**: So, thanks for joining us. Are you afraid to die?

**Rodney**: Wow, uh, whatever happened to opening with the easier questions; "What's your favorite color? What're the top songs on your iPod?"

**ENN**: Do you want to answer those questions?

**Rodney**: Well, I would've at least like to give a shout out to *The Police*, *U2* or *Vampire Weekend*.

**ENN**: You just did. Are you afraid to die?

**Rodney**: No, actually I'm not. That doesn't mean I'm ready for it to happen any time soon. As a matter of fact, I …

**ENN**: That's just a smokescreen, camouflage. When people say they aren't afraid to die—they just don't want to yet—it usually means they're very scared.

**Rodney**: I can't speak for others, even though I try to on my blog sometimes. I can just be as honest with myself as I know how to be and say no, I don't fear death.

**ENN**: Okay, we'll pretend you aren't lying. Why aren't you afraid to die?

**Rodney**: Oh, thank you *so much* for granting me leniency. I don't fear death because I feel deep within me that I was on another plane of existence before I joined this three-dimensional, earth-based one and that my soul will travel back to either that place before or a new place afterward.

**ENN**: You feel it? Do you have anything to back it up?

**Rodney**: Why, yes I do, but you're not going to like it.

**ENN**: Why is that?

**Rodney**: Because it's based on a mixture of science and faith and flowers. Are you ready?

**ENN**: Oh, do tell.

**Rodney**: Well, let's look at science for starters. The first law, the very first law of thermodynamics is what?

**ENN**: Energy can be changed but it can't be created or destroyed. Hey wait, we're the ones asking the questions. Why do you bring up the first law?

**Rodney**: It's self-explanatory, really. If some of the greatest scientific minds in the world hold this as their first law, who am I to blow against the wind?

**ENN**: Meaning?

**Rodney**: Meaning when you boil down our essence as humans, we are really just vast interconnections of love, thought, experience and learning. All those things are energy. How is it possible for that to vanish simply because we're closing our eyes for the final time on earth?

**ENN**: That sounds like mental gymnastics. What else do you have?

**Rodney**: Boy, you're tough. It really isn't gymnastics. When I think or when I dream or when I love, there are actual brainwaves that can be measured. You've seen the children's game at Toys R Us, haven't you? It allows you to manipulate a Star Wars object up and down just by thinking about it (*http://bit.ly/UXl5b3*) If you can buy something for $69.95(***batteries sold separately***) that's operated simply by brain activity, then mental gymnastics will only make me more hardy and fit.

**ENN**: Okay, you got me there. So we're energy ...

**Rodney**: Yes, and faith, too. But my faith is based on many things I've seen over the years and expect to keep seeing.

**ENN**: Such as?

**Rodney**: Well, coincidences, which aren't just incidents randomly happening at the same time. Then there are the deep emotional feelings suddenly springing out of the holy spots

I've experienced in the world. The feeling of my father's soul whooshing away as I held his dead body. The whole streetlights-talking-to-us thing. And lots more.

**ENN**: You realize that last paragraph was horrifically vague and rife with awkward grammar.

**Rodney**: Wow, if that's all you can respond with, I must be onto something. How about this: since the dawn of recorded history, there have always been deities among the lore and culture of societies. Sure, that shows there are always attempts to explain things with something other than pure cause and effect. But I have to believe there's something to the force that compels primitive societies, all the way up to today, to believe in something more out there.

**ENN**: Vague as can be.

**Rodney**: And yet you're interviewing me from something called "Eternity Network News."

**ENN**: Shush.

**Rodney**: Shush—how cosmic.

**ENN**: So you have a freakish admixture of faith and science going for you. Nice. What were you saying about flowers?

**Rodney**: I thought you'd forgotten. Flowers are just one of the many bits of proof for me that an overarching deity or a divine force exists in the universe.

**ENN**: "Deity"? "Divine Force"? Are you afraid to use the word "God"?

**Rodney**: Not at all. I just can't define what God means to me or to others. But there's no real explanation for flowers to be here or for them to be so brilliantly beautiful. Sure, you could say they evolved that way and they probably did. You could say they attract bees and the pollination process ensures their existence but many other plants need pollen and aren't nearly as pretty.

**ENN**: That's pretty shaky.

**Rodney**: Take it further. Why do we need lovely blossoms on this planet? Why do we need the bees that punch their time clocks at the flower factories? Why do we need the honey the bees make? Why do we need the bears that find that honey while out on a stroll with Christopher Robin? Why do we need anything other than strict functionality on earth? Keep going. Why do we need Earth?

**ENN**: You're getting out of control.

**Rodney**: No, it's simple. We don't need any of this when you take a strict, staunch scientific approach. None of this matters. The universe happened randomly; the Earth happened randomly; Cappuccino Blasts happened randomly. But I just can't believe deep in my soul that love, friendship, family, connections, kissing, great movies, emotions and pizza are just random occurrences that happened only because of the Big Bang.

**ENN**: Oh, so you believe in the Big Bang Theory? Do you believe in evolution too?

**Rodney**: Of course, but stay with me. Those two things—evolution and The Big Bang—explain what happened mechanically. I'm talking about what happened along with them as the systems progressed and what has happened in other galaxies and other planes of existence and …

**ENN**: Whoa, Rodney, hold on. You're just spouting off random spittle with no coherent thread.

**Rodney**: And you're about the worst interviewer I've ever met.

**ENN**: This story isn't going to lead tonight's newscast. I'd be surprised if it gets any play at all. So, how do you want it to end?

**Rodney**: Many years from now, frankly. And as a matter of fact, my doctor says all signs point to me living a long and healthy life.

**ENN**: This is definitely not getting any airtime. Anything else?

**Rodney**: Yeah, there is. Who are you really?

And with that, my three visitors ceremoniously remove their masks. We all burst out laughing and they speed-skate off this dimension to their live satellite truck on a shower of electrons and leave me wondering where to send my resume in 40 or 50 years.

CHAPTER **18**

# In My Room

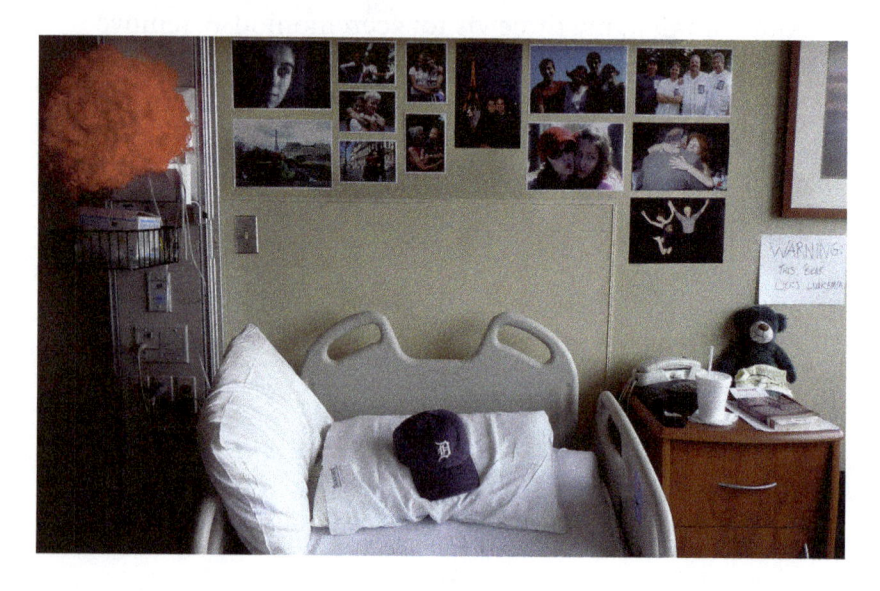

I HEAR IT'S hot.

Here, it's not.

This is the room with climate control.

My wallpaper is photos: girls, brothers, boys, a favorite nurse. My helmet is always near. So is my wig. My wig and helmet are the same, a soft hat from my cousin with an Olde English D.

An oxygen system is covered by another wig: a clown wig. You've seen me wear it for attention or diversion. You know it covers up nothing.

The doctor's hidden flashlight he forgot weeks ago nests in a basket near switches and plugs and medical things pretending to be oh-so-official. I've used the light to search for Mother Mary and God and Bodhisattvas and my dad.

This is the room with germ control.

I'm getting better in this room. *Up yours* to anyone who says otherwise. There are nights when I say *up yours* to yours truly.

There's a month in this room. There are the towels I've stuffed into the gaps between me and next door—a sometimes hospice room, sometimes healing. There's the bag of opened cards and the Nurses' Relief Station from my loving mom, full of candy.

There's a guy on a laptop. Who is he? I remember him when I see his eyes. I forget his silliness sometimes though. He sure was silly. God, was he fun.

Oh, oh, oh … he's poking his nose into the room.

This is the room where I control my mind, where I try to control my body.

Then the Beach Boys call to me from across time (*http://bit.ly/139v69X*) and even they're in my room.

**The Beach Boys - In My Room**

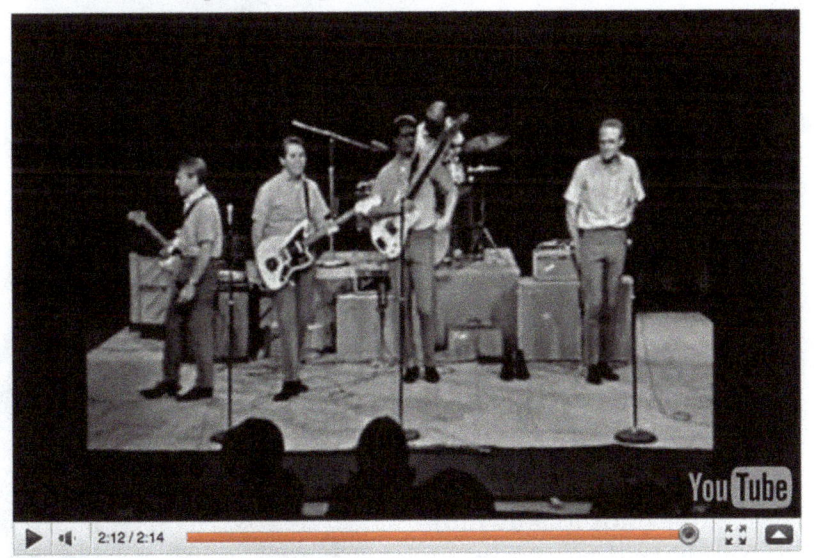

chapter 18 • 53

CHAPTER **19**

# Dreadlocks for Love

"Darrel, let me borrow your hair."

"What?"

"Come on, man, look at my bald scalp."

"He-he, Rodney … anything you say."

"Leslie, can you be the stylist?"

"Totally. Here, lay it like this."

"Gee, your hair smells terrific."

"Why, thank you, Rodney."

As my two dear friends leave, hope finds its way into my hospital room once more.

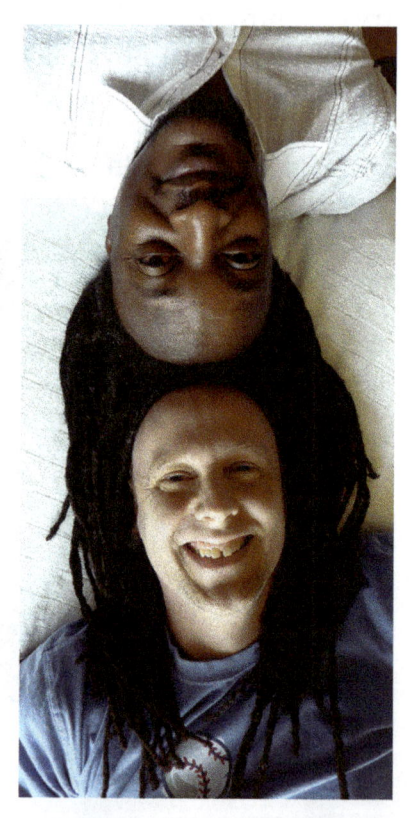

photo by Leslie Ellis

CHAPTER **20**

# Blimey, I'm in Rehab!

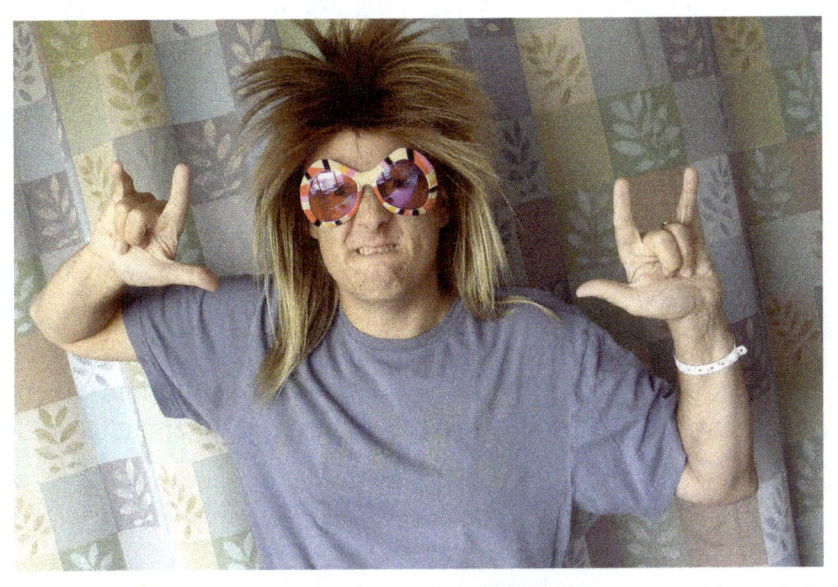

photo by J. Kyle Keener

FRIDAY AFTERNOON IS mellow. My doctor is pleased that my blood counts have flatlined (thank goodness I haven't), with all my numbers barely able to raise their hands for roll call. A hospital cheeseburger with fries is on the way.

Some photo friends show up with fun disguises and ...

And then suddenly I'm Nigel, an aging British rocker in rehab.

They're not photo friends anymore. Now they're my two longtime roadies who came to spring me. I sport an insane wig, Elton Gaga glasses and a tattoo saying either MOM or WOW, depending on how I affix it.

When Ronan and Aidan open the hermetically sealed items, my transformation is complete. No longer Rodney by the hour, I'm Nigel.

Dragging Ivy, my first stop is the nurses' station. A media frenzy ensues when they become the British tabloid press trying to do ol' Nigel in with their camera phones clicking and wanting to pose with me.

Several nurses who've treated me are now former lovers—that rapscallion Nigel has wronged them over the years. No one takes my suggestion seriously to slip a little gin or stout into my water cup.

Circling the ward with my phony-fake English accent, nurse Hellen becomes my beleaguered publicist, checking rooms for patients who'd remember me and my mates during our glam rock days. Then back in my private cell, I sink back into me.

There is a brief interruption when wife and daughter arrive and are rock-shocked by the getup, only to burst into insane laughter and pose on their own. So does my leukemia licker, now a hair bear.

Anyone who says life ain't grand, strongly needs a visit from their own private Nigel.

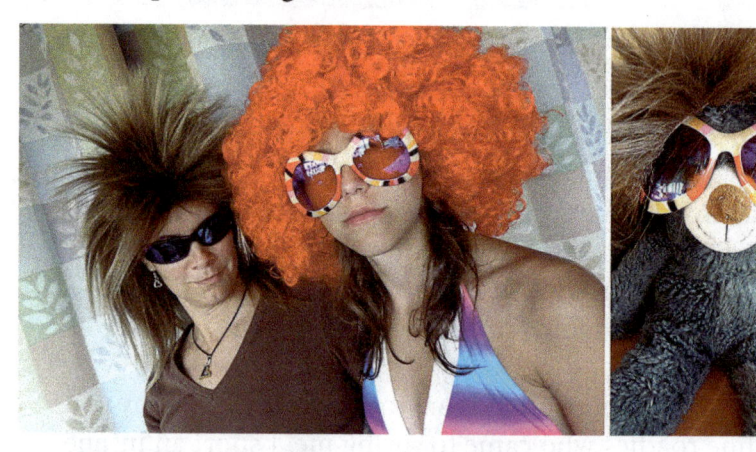

CHAPTER **21**

# $#%t

As the Rodney I once knew shrinks away in my hospital bed, I hope, pray and visualize great news in front of me. This morning I ran head-long into some lousy news.

The situation has taken a bit of a bad turn. It's not horrible, but nevertheless it's not the news I was looking for. This latest round of chemotherapy actually allowed for a slight increase of leukemia in my body. Can you imagine that; something called "high-dose Ara-C" actually let more cancer into my body? Now, it was only a *bit* more, but when you're thinking that maybe the news would be empty bones, it gets you even madder at the disease than the day before. Our family super hero, my Aunt-in-a-cape Roberta, speculates that the increase in cancer cells could be a false reading based on two different technical details. I'm hoping she's right.

So why did the cancer increase? Or did it? Nobody knows. Are there other options? Absolutely. It turns out there are chemotherapy cocktails my brand of leukemia hasn't even seen yet, and they promise to be devastating to the disease. Also, they are now scheduling me for bone marrow consultations. My brothers and cousins, as well as a vast sea of unknown persons, await donorship. One of them, if not one hundred, will be a match.

I still feel reasonably fine and healthy and my greatest advocates tell me my youth and health are vital to my treatments. My doctor has told his mentor, whom I'm scheduled to see, that when I walk into the room he won't believe I have leukemia (except maybe for my bald head).

I'm pissed. I despise leukemia more than ever. And I'm mad that my wife, daughters and mom have to go through this. They're handling it well, but I'm angry they even have something like this to "handle." Mom lost her own mother to cancer when she was 16. She lost her husband to cancer when she was 55. Her eldest had to have his thyroid obliterated due to, yep, cancer. Now me. No person should have to deal with that this many times.

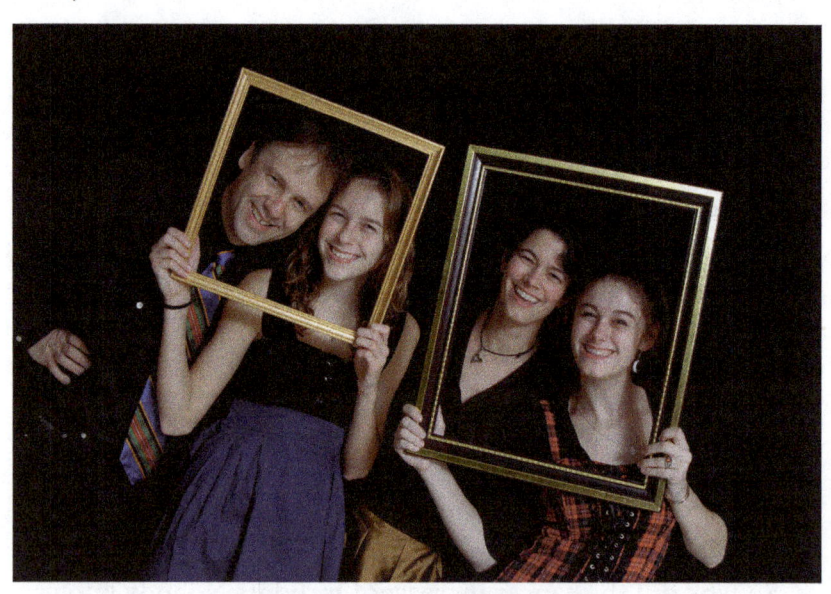

**photo by Leisa Thompson**

Am I thinking about the end game? Yes, but only in terms of a cure. Death is for a Rodney in his 80s or 90s. As Eminem says, "Success is my only mutherfuckin' option, failure's not." The Christmas picture we sent out last year, the one where we're all smiling and framed in portable frames, that's the image of my family I'm keeping. That's the one that will eventually eradicate cancer.

My climb just became a bit steeper. I would be lying if I said otherwise. My prognosis is still for a cure and not just remission. They're sending me home for a few days, too. My own bed and family will comfort me until I report back for duty.

Mom always said with bad news comes good.

CHAPTER **22**

# Home

IT'S BEEN A very scattered, yet relaxing, time away from the front lines. Sleep is my biggest luxury. I can't explain why sleeping in the hospital is so tough; it should be the number one easiest thing. Everyone since Hippocrates (*http://bit.ly/139v6a0*) has said sleep is one of the body's most important defenses.

Back there, in *that* place, my night nurses would sometimes "Q-shift" me, meaning they'd check my vital signs once at the beginning of the shift and once at the end. Barring any night noises, interruptions, beepings, buzzings or people emptying my trash at 0-dark thirty, it usually meant I'd be able to sleep an hour or two before the constant drip from my gal-pal Ivy sent me to the toilet.

The past several nights at home, I've gotten 7-8 hours at a stretch, then a few more ... then some more. Home life is a posh existence.

Marci and I went down to the Karmanos Cancer Institute to up the ante in this war on leukemia. They seem to love anomalies and eat them for breakfast. If my genes are screwed up, or if I should want or require experimental treatments, they're ready like Igor and Dr. F to jump in. I don't actually know when I'll be inserted into their system, but the myriad vials of blood they sucked out of me indicate they're arming themselves for battle.

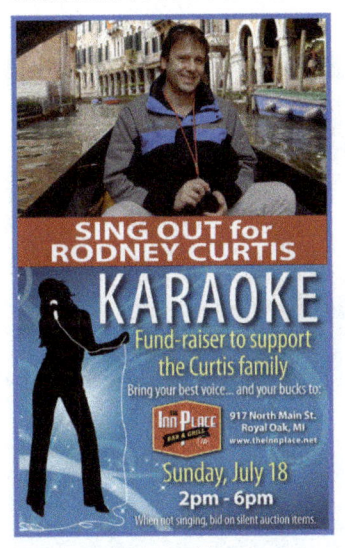

There's an incredible karaoke fundraiser going on tomorrow at The Inn Place in Royal Oak (*http://bit.ly/VN2Vbi*). It was organized by a dude who was laid off the same time as me, Marty Westman, with a helping hand from the amazing Sally Tato Snell. Both are so modest, I can't actually tell who did what.

"So, how are you doing, Rodney?" is the number one question I hear continually. And yes, I'm happy to answer. I don't really feel like I have cancer or anything other than the easy fatigue that hovers right nearby. I know I'm in the middle of an enormous fight and these brutal cells inside me just aren't agreeing to a ceasefire. I appreciate the thousands of well-wishes I'm getting from friends as distant as elementary school and as recent as my new hospital buddies. The only thing separating me from that dude riding the gondola in Marty's poster is a head of hair and, well, that sexy silhouette.

I have more things written out and stacked up, ready to land like planes at Detroit Metro, but I thought I'd just toss out a little of this, a little of that tonight. Now it's back to my insanely soft couch, followed by my one-of-a-kind bed. Know this; know this from every clean and clear cell in my body: I am going to rid leukemia from my lifestyle and come back as the kind of person I've always known I can be.

chapter 22 • 61

CHAPTER **23**

# A Funraiser

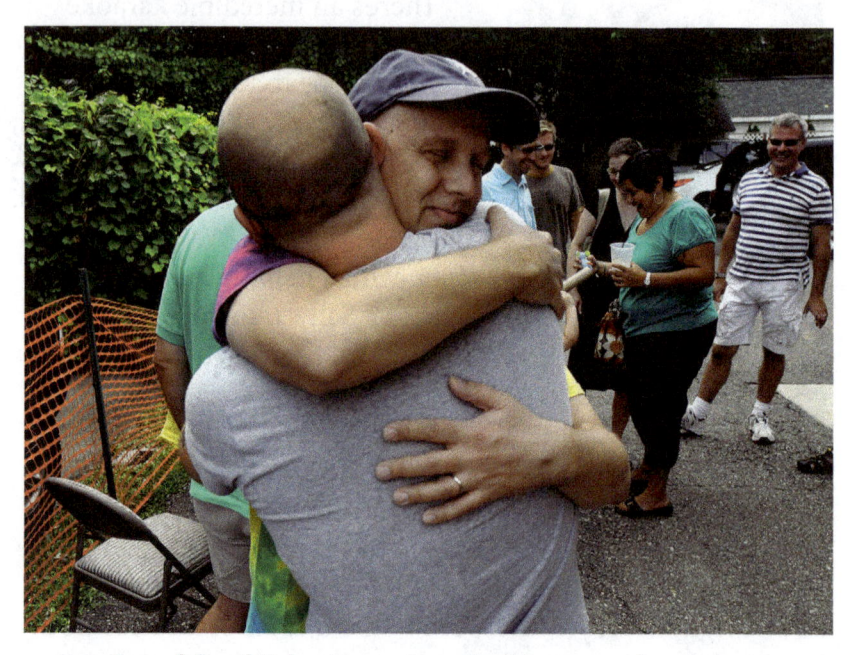

*I give old pal Tyler Rau a hug in this marvelous photo shot by Stephen Perez at the fundraiser in my name.*

Hey, quick show of hands. How many of you think coincidences are simply random, unrelated events? One ... two ... maybe three of you.

Great, okay, how many of you know in your gut that coincidences signify something more, but you just can't figure it out? Whoa ... OK, one, two, three, four, five, six, seven, eight, nine ... got it. And that's just the first row of you. I see.

Something amazing happened Sunday afternoon. If you're thinking it was all the love, outflowing of support, amazing acts of kindness from strangers and a festival of genuine friendship, then you're mostly right. But there was something else buried in the bar. I'll get to that in a moment, but first a confession.

I was nervous. I was very, very nervous. I didn't even know how apprehensive I was until I stood there, outside a fundraiser thrown together to help my family pay our cancer bills. I was talking to friends and realized my knees were actually shaking. If you feel like attributing it to chemotherapy and a general, overall fatigue, be my guest. But the honest emotion coursing through me at that moment was an anxiety for what was happening all around me.

Goodness knows I love the spotlight. I can't tell you how much I love things being all about me. But Sunday's silent auction and karaoke event brought out an aspect of me I didn't realize existed. I didn't know what to expect. I felt weird showing up with my bald head conspicuously covered with a Detroit Tigers cap. I didn't know who in the world would want to give up their gorgeous, sunny Sunday afternoon to hang out in a dark bar and sing old songs. I was—okay I'll say it—afraid.

I feared no one would show up. I feared being stared at. I feared people would think I was trying to use cancer as a way to make money. I feared I'd have no stamina. I feared x, y and z.

Then, I just accepted it all. I accepted the person I never met who made a cool, retro ice chest which made a handsome decoration and a handsome profit. I accepted all the amazing photos which were fiercely bid upon. I accepted the photo lamp and the fishing trip and the karaoke singers, and the, and the, and the, from people who knew me well, knew me a little or didn't know me at all.

Accepting charity is normally very hard for me. Each person there made it simple.

There are so many organizers to thank, from the guy who got laid off the same day I did, to the owners of The Inn Place (*http://bit.ly/VN2Vbi*) where it was held,

chapter 23 • 63

to everyone who just came to have some fun. It was my mom, though, who felt most like a celebrity when so many people came over and had a kind word for me or her. It made her week, or even her month.

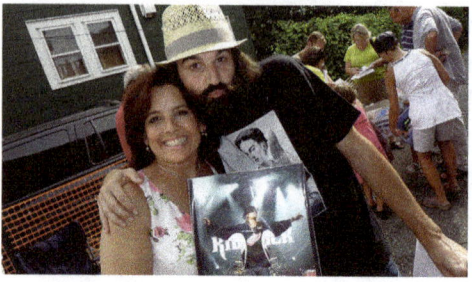

**Cheryl Webster Miller won one of Romain Blanquart's photos of Kid Rock**

So ... coincidences, right? Only a few people are aware of this, but a day earlier, when Marci and I met with the Karmanos Cancer Institute team to determine our next course of attack, they told us our insurance probably wouldn't cover bone marrow testing for my cousin and brothers—the likeliest of donor matches. Through a crazy loophole, which is being closed by the blessed Obama health care plan, our insurer, HAP, can deny payment for their tests, but will allow unrelated searches through an anonymous registry. As ridiculous as that sounds, there's a scenario that could've led to us owing a large chunk of money.

Yes, a very large chunk of money indeed. That amount was so large that it actually made us begin to question how we'd handle the search and maybe we'd try this or that to cut back.

That amount was a mountain.

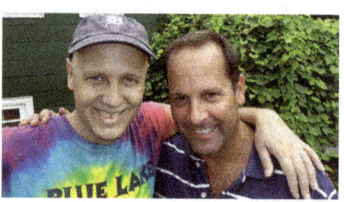

**I get to partially thank Marty Westman**

Yet that amount was slid into a shopping bag, donated throughout the day by friends and strangers, then handed to Marci and me before we drove away.

That exact amount.

There were many other coincidences, both major and minor. Without explaining myself, if you're ever in the Detroit area, you should definitely try Shield's pizza (*http://bit.ly/ TV339o*). I owe karma that little plug. Don't worry if you don't buy into the coincidences-as-something-more philosophy. Coincidences don't get hurt feelings.

As we took off down Main St., my bride of 20 years asked, "So, how do you feel?" And then her laughter slipped and slid out as I sat in the passenger seat, open-mouthed without a sound coming out. For the first time since she's known me, I was left speechless.

CHAPTER **24**

# Golden Bubbles and Silver Linings

**THERE'S SOMETHING STIRRING** inside **of me**. Please forgive me if I talk in circles here, but something is happening and I'm trying to find the proper way to explain it.

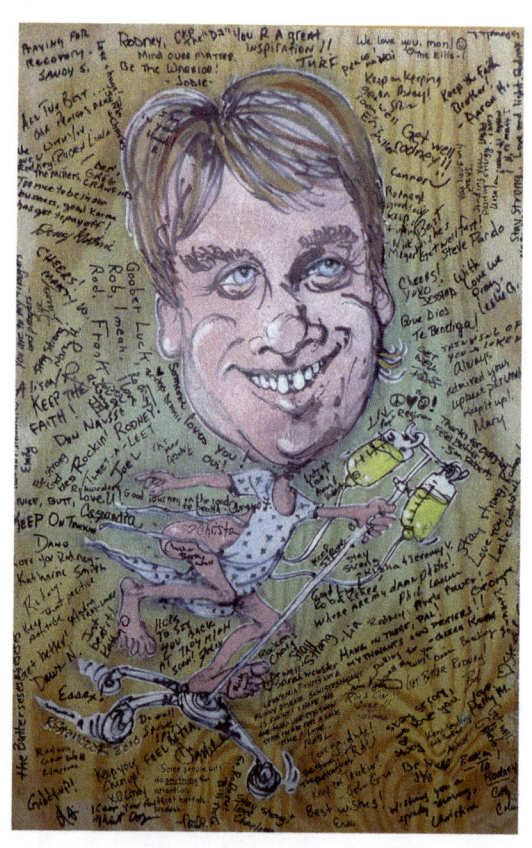

Graphic artist Ray Stanczak created this wooden wonder of me, which everyone signed with wishes of wellness.

**I began to notice a stirring inside of me** on Sunday, the day we spent visiting our daughters at Blue Lake Fine Arts Camp (*http://bit.ly/VN2Vbl*) and attending an extraordinary fundraiser. My eldest, Skye, led me through a mind-over-matter exercise, after we had lunch that day. It involved golden bubbles coursing through me, gently easing good white blood cells into existence and ushering the naughty ones away. Later that day, "coincidentally," a fellow survivor wrote a serious note on a silly caricature of me. "Rodney, mind over matter," he said.

My daughter's internal visualization began to take hold, fertilized by the love and buoyant support surrounding me at that fundraiser. Inward changes fostered by outward buttressing. That's a potent mix. Wait, I think I've got it. Let me begin this a third and final time.

**Something wonderful is stirring deep within me.** Yes. That's it. There's something wonderful within. A routine blood test this week, the kind you sometimes hear about on "Grey's Anatomy," revealed certain levels of certain counts to be twice as high as back when I was "healthy" a year ago. My doctor didn't believe the test. He thought his machine was broken. A second test told him they were real.

He apparently hasn't witnessed golden bubbles or karaoke fundraisers or mind messing with matter. My treatment plans are now in a tizzy. No one exactly knows which end is up. A fourth plug of marrow will soon be removed from my hips, which have become so comfortable with the procedure, that when they see the needle and corkscrew, they just yawn, roll sideways and flip on an old "Seinfeld" rerun.

When you look at our year, there hasn't been a lot to cheer about. And yet there are so many positives that have sprung out of the negatives, as my mother has always told me. Being unemployed gave me a lot of time with the family and allowed me the luxury of heading to the hospital on that Sunday evening in April to have my gall bladder examined. Had there been a job the following morning, I would've waited the extra

chapter 24 • 67

five or 10 minutes for the gut pain to subside, (which it did), then headed off to bed. That Rodney guy wouldn't have found out his white blood cells were dangerously low. Being unemployed also presented me with the opportunity to teach some college classes, something I always thought I'd be good at. Turns out, I was mostly right about that.

The car accident that totaled our van while Marci waited at the stoplight turned positive when it took our 12-year-old van with 180,000 miles and replaced it with a 10-year-old van with only 80,000 miles.

The money stolen from our locked safe in Paris was reimbursed by the hotel management. And it gave us a chance to speak with the *gendarmes*, Interpol and feel like we were part of any given spy film from the past decade.

The new start-up newspaper, which closed after only five days, saved me mountains of headaches due to extreme underfunding.

And as Marci said, after nudging me in bed, "Your leukemia is bringing out the best in people." She's right. Armies of friends and strangers are committing acts of such brazen kindness, it almost feels illegal to enjoy the fruits of their offerings. Even though our family is insured, people still muscle their way to the front of the line and offer up newer and more creative ways to help out.

My cousin Chris explained that people need to do good and I am giving them the opportunity to do so. As I bumble through this cancer experience, I sometimes think—but only for a moment—that might be part of my role. No, I'm not so arrogant as to imply it's because of my disease that all my friends are being awesome. That doesn't explain it. But try this t-shirt on for size: by swallowing my pride and allowing others to do nice things, I am letting a greater good metastasize around me. Each one of you does good every day. Just seeing it all happen in one confined location is simply astounding.

**Something is stirring outside of me now.**

CHAPTER **25**

# Peter's Principles

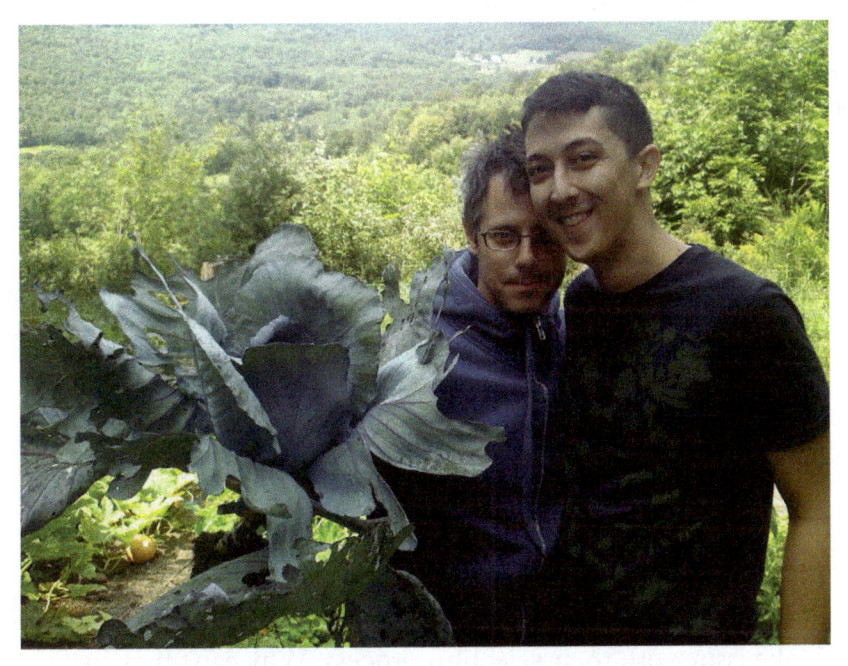

Pictured, from left to right: A cabbage, Peter, then Masood. Photo by Peter Ross.

ON SEPTEMBER 11<sup>TH</sup>, after both twin towers were hit, I called my buddy Peter to find out what was happening. Peter lived in lower Manhattan at the time and my little paper in Midland (*http://bit.ly/VN2SfL*) was like every other news organization, trying to make sense of the madness. Peter's partner, Masood, got on the line and gave us some good, solid quotes about what he was witnessing.

That wasn't the first time I asked Peter for help. Nor would it be the last. I had already known him for 14 years and trusted him as a journalist, photographer (*http://bit.ly/TV350P*) and friend. He and I met at the exact same time that Marci and I met at the now-defunct *Ann Arbor News*. I remember a conversation, which in retrospect, is hilarious. I told Peter I was interested in Marci and hopefully he wouldn't mind if I continued trying to get into her good graces.

Peter didn't mind at all. I found out later, through a great multi-page, handwritten letter, that he was gay.

Back then it wasn't as easy to be "out." These days it hardly seems to be an issue. The ABC Family network has gay teen characters and my daughters know many openly homosexual kids in middle school and high school.

But there are still places and institutions where it's not easy being gay in this country. Apparently one of those places is the bone marrow donor program. Peter, who gave me that bright clown wig, who I've counted on for almost two dozen years, who is nothing but amazing, was rejected due to sexual orientation. He tried to donate, but they told him they were concerned about HIV. Peter doesn't have HIV. Lots of straight folks have HIV, however.

I feel rotten about that. The marrow program will be one of the factors that cures me. It will make sure leukemia stays far away and doesn't rear its ugly head after two or 20 years. But I take issue with their selection process. Why can't they just screen Peter's test like they do everyone else's? If people are being excluded, doesn't it just naturally follow that potential recipients are losing out?

I'm not on a crusade here. I'm just a guy hopefully recovering from cancer who thinks a lot more people could benefit if the gene pool were expanded. I'm no clinician or researcher and I certainly don't understand actuarial tables. If someone wants to selflessly give of themselves, shouldn't they be allowed to do so?

Maybe I should be silent and not cause waves. I wouldn't want the program's upper echelon to catch wind of my friend's rejection or my feelings of injustice. I need their marrow. It would be reckless or feckless to openly ask for an explanation.

I guess I'm just not the silent type.

CHAPTER **26**

# Remission Accomplished

I'M LOOKING FOR allegories and metaphors in this rabid rainstorm sweeping across our viewing area. Is it a cleansing, soothing rain that wipes away the past, or is it more a reminder of the spectacular power all around us? It bends trees to the breaking point but they sway back into place. The lightning scares away the shadows for an instant and the thunder is so loud and near that my very marrow shakes.

My very marrow shakes.

Was that an accidental analogy or did the thunder clap shake it free? And what was the real thunder clap? Was it the deep rumble that just shook the house or the simple declaration, repeated three, four, 20 times by my doctor, *"You are in remission."*

Listen to that echo: remission ...remission ...remission ...

Listen to the storm subside.

Listen to Peter Gabriel singing "Solsbury Hill" over and over and over again as I wait for my family to arrive to hear about my sweet marrow. My lovely bones. My family will laugh as they recall my eating ribs for good luck the other night. They'll mob me and cry. They may even rub my scalp whiskers for continued luck.

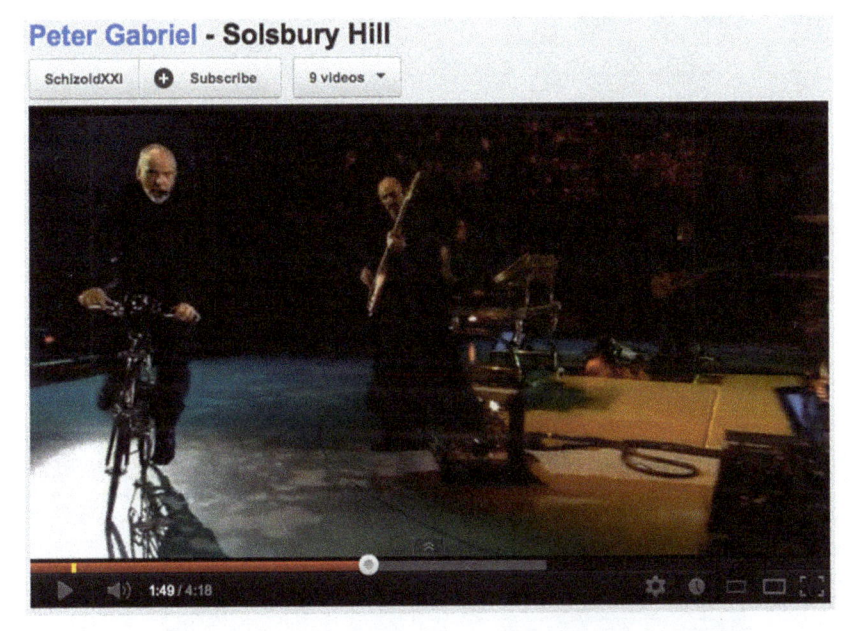

**There is joy and wonder in our family-favorite, Peter Gabriel's Solsbury Hill (http:bit.ly/UXmcl1).**

The dogs will bark. My friends will start to wonder about my chest tubes and more chemo and practical/important things that friends need to wonder about. I'll explain there's more chemotherapy ahead, but in manageable doses meant to perma-smack leukemia back where it came from and beyond. I'll mention, casually, that we still don't know what's up with the marrow transplant thing, then I'll thank them for being so caring.

Wait. That's the garage door. That's them.

Dancing, hopping and hoping, hugging like World Series champs, tears, barking, laughing, disbelief, re-belief, everything.

Look at the blue sky now.

God, Shiva, Mohammed, Buddha, Jesus, Mary, Dad ... look at that blue, blue sky now.

CHAPTER 27

# I Have a What the Size of a What, Where?

YOU CAN TAKE the cancer out of the man, but you can't take the man out of the hospital, apparently. Maybe I should start with why I've been sitting in a Muskegon hospital for the better part of three days.

My extended family had been planning a trip to our favorite Lake Michigan location. I went to summer camp near here for four years, the girls go to Blue Lake Fine Arts Camp near here, we've rented cottages from numerous people since back when a week on the lake cost about $300, and we all just love to relax and plop down and think about nothing for a while. There's no cell service, no Internet, and I think the TV may get "I Love Lucy," but nobody has flipped it on.

I spent the week before the drive up congested. It was knocking me down something fierce and I would have to take baby steps, relax, a few more baby steps, then maybe nap. It kind of seemed to me like *that* was how leukemia was supposed to feel. A couple of my oncologists looked me over but just prescribed some more cold medicine and I was off to the cottage.

The first night there, though, before everyone else showed up, I had "The Incident." I woke up unable to breathe and alerted the rest of the darkened place by pounding the walls, floors and even the door as I lurched out into the kitchen. Big brother Dean, from California, grabbed hold of me and was able to hear me say "water."

Somehow in his arms I was able to exhale. Maybe I was able to breathe all along and had only been trying to inhale, but to say that moment was one of the most frightening of my life would be an understatement. A little water and a late night phone call to a third oncologist helped ease the situation.

The next morning, on the long-distance advice of my Aunt-in-a-cape Roberta, my brother Dean drove me down to a Muskegon emergency room and, after switching hospitals on me due to procedures, it turns out I have, (or *had* at this point), "an impressive blood clot, the size of a half-eaten hot dog."

The amazing Doctor Mallon has spent the last two or three days pounding the clot, which rested near my heart, with a series of chemicals and then a tiny balloon and then something I referred to as sort of a carpet cleaner (he liked the analogy). It wasn't the exact way I thought of spending my vacation, a tour of Muskegon hospitals, but they are very impressive over here on this side of the state.

He said cancer drugs and this large medical port inside of me were to blame for the blood clot; it was nothing I did or didn't do.

Lying prone in the ICU, I look at the positives ... at least I have web access. This hospital wireless service seems strong and solid, far more so than me. They are going to release me to spend a day or two longer at the cottage, then it's back to Troy and my newest round of chemo beginning on Monday.

But through all of this—well, most of it anyway—there has been an acute awareness that I'm in remission and whatever life feels the need to throw at me, it's okay. I was kind of wondering how this whole cancer experience would change me and there, right there, seems to be one of the core fundamental shifts. Let's see if it's real or lasts.

I can do without the late night scary bits though.

CHAPTER **28**

# What Lies Ahead

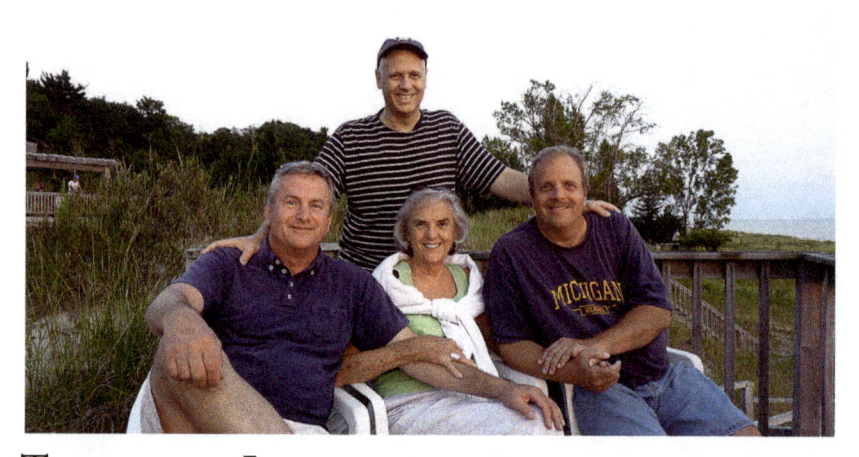

**TOMORROW I CHECK** into the hospital for my next round of chemo. I don't fear it though, I spent half an hour in Jo-Ann Fabrics (*http://bit.ly/TV339s*) this morning and after that, any form of torture—medical or medieval—doesn't faze me one bit.

After being sprung from the Muskegon Clot-Busters Palace, I once again entered the health system to continue my sojourn toward wellness, productivity and a full head of hair. In between last week and now, though, were several wonderful hours relaxing at Lake Michigan with my family and about four or five minutes of intense go-kart racing where, if Taylor is to be believed, my daughter and her cousin left me in their distant exhaust. There's something about remission that makes my family not treat me with kid gloves anymore. I'll say it: she should've let me win.

This, in some ways, becomes the boring part of my saga. Sure, the questions loom large about my eventual outcome—marrow replacement or just tons more chemo. The small scheduling scenarios also come into play—will I stay in the hospital after the treatment or come home to recuperate? Can the family count on me for the first day of school or all the intense last-of-summer ballyhoos? What about the fall weddings I'm supposed to shoot?

The latter has been answered, or at least the pressure has been alleviated by two wonderful brides I've never met. They have both sent me exceptionally warm wishes and said they'll accept whatever I can do. If I need one of my many super-duper-shooter friends to help me, that's fine by them. If I can do it myself, great. If someone else has to shoot it solo, sure Rodney, no problem.

When it comes to the rest of the unknowns, honestly, I'm a journalist by training and thus have an incredibly high tolerance for ambiguity. I used to preach that to my interns or to whoever would listen. Trust that things will fall into place and the feeling in your gut right now will very soon be less knotted and more at ease.

I obviously need that very advice right now.

Since I always try to be honest with myself, I don't feel I've adequately or fully dealt with the emotions surrounding cancer and the unexpected half-eaten hotdog that was lurking next to my heart. Sure I've cried and laughed and talked and thought about it all, but I think there's a longer answer ahead of me. I know there are deeper discoveries about myself just waiting to be spelunked. And I completely believe, with every paisley Jo-Ann fabric of my being, that I'm coming out of this experience changed for the better.

I'd like to reiterate something that has been laughing and bouncing around me for about as long as the cancer's been poking sharp sticks at me. The interconnections that we all share may not seem significant now, as you sit in health and normalcy. But please know, when the ride starts to get scary, there are people you haven't even met out there—as well as your closest friends—who will jump into the seat next to you and help keep you calm, secure, fed and smiling. You don't always know it until you need it, but those bridges you didn't burn years ago will allow your past to come visit your present.

And if you were truly good to your past, they'll bring snacks.

CHAPTER 29

# Messing With the Messengers

THE PRIEST POKED his head inside my hospital room again, looked down at his notes and stared back at me with a blank expression. Apparently I wasn't Catholic enough for him. He always looks at me confused. It stems back to the time when he offered me a prayer and I stupidly said, "Sure, from which spiritual vantage point?"

The notes in his hand didn't really carry a good answer. I asked him for something from Zarathustra and he smiled slowly, then boogied quickly.

I sometimes get that way in normal life, testing people who come at me trying to sell a political candidate, a new church, or gutter cleaning. Salespeople showing up at your door probably despise having to ring doorbells. I should be nicer. Here in the hospital they aren't allowed to sell roofing services or premium cable connections, but I get a nice mix of God's salespeople stopping by my chemo lair.

Another Catholic priest who popped into my room recently offered me communion. I was game; it had been a while since

I'd gone through the ceremony. But moments before he offered up the piety pita for my consumption, I casually mentioned I wasn't—in fact—Catholic. I didn't really like the look in his eye as he glanced from me to his notes and back.

"Aren't you _____?" he asked.

When I told him *blank* didn't live here anymore, he ended the interchange. I didn't realize it was Canon Law to refuse communion to those not technically Catholic. Besides, I shoot with Nikons.

Now this much I do know: I've taken communion in a Catholic church on at least two separate occasions without being given a Spanish Inquisition (of course, *nobody* expects the Spanish Inquisition (*http://bit.ly/TV350V*)). Then again, those were times in my youth when one of my many Catholic friends had to attend church on Saturday night or Sunday and I was having a sleepover with them so I just went along for the righteous ride. One awkward incident happened in high school when my buddy Bob and I were on vacation and he found a remote church along Lake Michigan to attend.

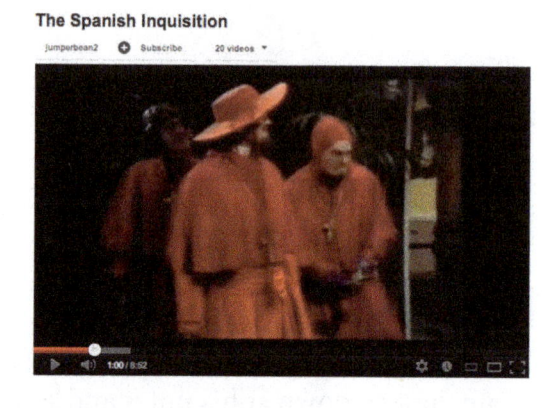

"Okay, Bob, I'm doing everything you do. I take the holy wafer in my hand, then I accept the drink, then later we hug the hot chicks in the pews and say 'Peace Be With You,' right? I'll kneel when you do and say 'trespasses' instead of 'debts.' Anything else?"

Bob said I'd covered all the bases. Then we walked into the small clapboard church and he suddenly makes a gesture with the birdbath inexplicably placed right inside the door and wipes his hand off on his shirt a few times, then his forehead.

82 • A "Cute" Leukemia

Uhhh, okay, so I did the same thing, using my shirt and pants though.

To this day I don't know if he just forgot to tell me about blessing yourself with holy water as you enter a church or if he simply wanted to see how I'd react.

Another monotheistic misstep occurred when a substitute minister entered my hospital room and was sweet, caring, full of smiles and couldn't get my name right to save her soul (okay, not a good sentence to use that cliché). She asked if she could say a prayer for me and I gladly agreed. Closing my eyes, she lit into a fabulous prayer about health and vitality and love, all for "Randy." She must've thought I was a fool, sitting there laughing my head off. But it was a very kind and heartfelt prayer so I forwarded it mentally to two different Randys I know who have cancer. No need letting such a prayer go to waste. I hope you received it, Randys. Remember to recycle.

Thank God the hospital has Reverend Rik. He's the official cancer ward Soul Man and I defy you to spend two minutes in his company and not see a being of light and love. Mostly, Rik is the type of reverend who gives spirituality a great name, doesn't push it down your throat and is just as comfortable talking about silly things on the Internet as he is about God, Jesus and hospital food. Rik's the real deal and we are all lucky to have him out there.

For me, a guy who bills himself as a "Spiritual Wanderer," the last thing I want to do is ice out or write off religions I don't agree with—although I'm not a fan of the Taliban's way of practicing their political spirituality. Reading this over, I hope you don't get the impression that I'm mocking certain faiths. I just enjoy poking fun at myself and sometimes I take others along for the ride with me.

In the words of a dearly departed Rodney, "Can we all get along?"

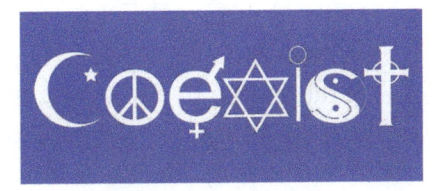

CHAPTER **30**

# Ends and Odds

**ONE OF THE** mind excursions I used back when I didn't have a handle on leukemia was to think about the long-term future. I'd fantasize about anything I could Velcro my soul to. That way, if I cemented a future far enough ahead, I was sure to move toward it, as opposed to slipping into the muck of the moment or worse, watching CNN and worrying about the larger things I couldn't control.

∼

**My favorite future flight of fantasy:** I'm rolling in the grass next to our home, years and years down the road, with one of my daughter's kids. We laugh, get dirty, then flip onto our backs and look up at the clouds.

Pointing up at a thick, robust cumulus I ask, "Do you know what that cloud's called?"

Without missing a beat, my grandchild answers, "Marvin."

We laugh like hyenas, then notice my wife over in the tall grass, pulling out weeds and we instantly become lions stalking our prey. As we move closer to the lone animal, separated from her herd, I realize that absolutely no good will come from the scenario, but I'm powerless to stop the slaughter.

**Attitude's everything:** Every single doctor, nurse, clinician and dietician I run into tells me a positive mental attitude is the number one key to beating disease. I'm glad to hear that but I also know cancer has become so much less of a death sentence these days than it was even 10 years ago. I can't tell you the number of people that have said, "Oh, my sister/wife/husband/sous-chef had cancer and is completely cured, living an exciting life."

**The most outrageous mistake I made with my jumbled up chemo-brain:** I was telling my cousin, niece and sister-in-law about the bone marrow donor questions we had. I informed them, "Yes, we're looking for a perfect boner donor."

**The most competitive I've ever felt while going through a medical procedure:** When I was in the Muskegon hospital operating room and the funny Dr. Mallon was prodding my veins with a plastic line to destroy the blood clot, he asked if I knew any jokes. My mind dug up some of my bluer material and I laid one on him. He countered with something just as risqué. (Two female nurses were snickering in the room, by the way.) I hit him with another, he retaliated. By the time we got up to about five or six jokes each, I was feeling the effects of the anesthesia and had to back out gracefully.

He won that round, beating both my humor and my blood clot.

CHAPTER **31**

# Is the Patient In?

A SHORT TAP-TAPPING at the door occurs as I'm leaving my room to make the mile lap around the ward. A couple candy-stripers with "The Cart" peek in. From The Cart you can purchase chocolate, salty snacks, little games, weekly news magazines or maybe some illicit drugs if you know the right code words.

You can't get Belgian beer or pizza from The Cart, I've checked.

The two young ladies, hardly 20, look at me and then look back into my room and ask, "Is the patient here? He may want to buy something."

Moments later, the nurses on the ward comment on how fast I'm walking those laps and how big the smile on my face looks.

CHAPTER **32**

# Blood Brothers

I DIDN'T KNOW why my big brother Scott was leaning across the ripped vinyl seats in our 1970s station wagon. He had a goofy smile plastered across his face. But when he pushed up against me and buried his mouth and nose in my chest, I knew in my nine-year-old mind I shouldn't fear getting hit. From there, muffled by my shirt, I heard him sing, "Come on people now, smile on your brother." (*http://bit.ly/TV350X*)

He was actually doing that, smiling on his brother.

Neither of us really understood how to smile on someone, or what the song actually meant. But he took the initiative and gave it a whirl in the back of our puke-yellow car with the impossibly garish, fake wood decals along the side. I give him credit for trying.

My relationship with Scott has always been a sociologist's dream. He was the youngest in the family for six years until I bumbled out of the womb and spoiled his streak. Securing the role of middle child, he fought equally hard against Dean, our oldest, and me. The battles with Dean were epic, as the two were pretty evenly matched, being only 14 months apart. One time, I showed up in their bedroom and heard pounding and yelling. Somehow Dean had shoved Scott into their closet and jammed the door shut with a spare crutch leftover from the time Dean's plan to karate kick the medicine cabinet door didn't exactly work out as planned.

Scott's battles with me were more like the Nazis invading Poland, only I didn't have the international community in an uproar over my beatings. Surrender was my only option.

I always knew Scott had my back though. The neighborhood bullies didn't seem to come by for a second round of mayhem at my expense once he paid them a visit. And I can distinctly remember a long-ago adventure in the park at the end of our street, next to the chemical factory. The place was packed and my big brother was actually a bit shaken up when he thought he'd lost me to the crowd of kids who'd gathered in the summer night to watch somebody do something—lost to time— invariably wrong or illegal.

As we got older though, a real respect for each other began to take hold and—shock upon shock—we found out we actually enjoyed being in each other's company. Whereas we used to pass the time goading each other until Mom or Dad yelled at us (usually yelling at him because I played the victim card **all** the time), now we golf. He still beats me though, only now it's with the number of swings it takes to put the damn ball in the cup.

I'd say we've progressed up the socially acceptable ladder a rung or two.

When I got tackled by leukemia a few months ago, I could see the pain in my big brother's eyes. I don't know this for a fact, but it seemed to me they were saying, "Come on Rodney, how am I supposed to protect you from *this*?"

He's often stopped by my hospital room or swung by the house and mowed my lawn for me. He's done what he could, lifting my spirits, talking about the Tigers, telling jokes, having his bone marrow tested, that sort of thing.

We've known throughout this disease that my prognosis, if everything goes according to plan, is very good. We've also witnessed things not going at all according to plan. For the past several weeks we've been on the course from remission to a cure by doing more chemotherapy and knocking leukemia completely and totally out of me forever.

The best way to do that, we're told, is by replacing my bone marrow with someone else's. Several people have been tested, including my brothers and a cousin and there have even been folks in the national registry, friends of mine, who've sent me their anonymous code numbers in case we were a match.

A couple days ago, one of those anonymous numbers hit. I was told I won the lottery. It was actually my brother Scott's marrow, which at this point looked like a perfect match for my own. He had been in the national registry years earlier for a firefighter friend of his and due to our similar genetic makeup, he appeared to be the perfect donor for me. In the crass words of a couple buddies 30 years ago, "You and your brother are fucking clones."

My creative brother figured out yet another way to smile on me.

"So Scott, how are you feeling today?" I asked when I phoned him. "How do your bones feel?" I told him the news and he was extremely happy for me, and I think a bit for himself too. Upon further conversation, when he learned all he had to do was basically just give blood and not go under the knife or pickaxe or corkscrew, he seemed even happier.

He was happier still when I agreed that a meal at Ruth's Chris Steakhouse (*http://bit.ly/VN2Vbs*) would be the perfect way to prep his blood for sharing. The dude's giving me his stem cells; the least I can do is order him a filet or something.

CHAPTER **33**

# Next to Normal

I**N MY HOSPITAL** stays so far—with this disease and the freaky blood clot over in Muskegon—I've craved lots of different things. I was on a pizza jag for a while, then burgers. Pepsi Slurpees have always filled the bill and an occasional caramel shake has been delivered by my ever supportive family. But the growing, all-consuming craving I'm experiencing these days is for normalcy.

(With a side of fries.)

I know I've given normalcy a bad rap sometimes in my life. There were times I've felt if things are normal, I'm not growing or expanding my horizons. Sure, it sounds pathologic, but I used to fear contentment. I distinctly remember a conversation with a long-ago girlfriend where I said, "If I start talking about end tables, just kill me."

Yes, I eventually capitulated and now I have an end table. But back then it seemed so grown up, so settled, so usual, so normal. Now I crave normal. I crave my own bed. I crave not walking around with tubes coming out of me. I crave not having to schedule time to see my family. I even crave mowing the lawn.

I was moments away from getting a day pass out of this hospital last week to go see my daughter's marching band show, and at the last minute they rescinded it. I'm a grown man asking the teacher for a pass to walk the hallways. It feels so out of my control and yet I know all of this is for a great reason, my health.

But it's going to be a while before I see normal again.

First my brother has to give me his stem cells. Even though they still call it marrow donation, they aren't actually going and taking his bone marrow. Instead they extract stem cells, just like you're giving blood and then whisk it over to me where it'll just drip intravenously into my Red River.

They will give me even more chemo beforehand, then the recovery process begins with several more weeks in the hospital. Then there could be years of anti-rejection precautions and crazy things like getting all my baby shots redone since I have a brand new system.

I'm looking at normal occurring sometime, I just don't know when.

But will it ever be normal? Is this the new normal? Will I be able to go on vacation again and not fear waking up in the middle of the night with a blood clot? Or will my new normal include a perspective that I normally don't have?

Will I be thankful for every day and treat those around me with a greater abundance of respect and admiration? Will I look at this as a second chance and an opportunity to get things right? Or will I be so thankful for normalcy that I'll just sink back into old roles and not feel affected by the shadow of cancer in my past?

These are all the random ramblings of a guy who's been hospitalized far too much this summer, so take them with a grain of salt substitute. I know my future holds change and growth and an appreciation far greater than I've ever experienced. But from the viewpoint of a gray hospital morning, that future looks vague and distant.

And then a large family walks, heads bowed, out of a darkened patient's room a few doors down. Their faces show incomprehension—the telltale signs the end is near—and I feel like a jerk. Here I am, hinting towards healthy and their options have run out.

Thank God I *have* a vague and distant future.

CHAPTER **34**

# To the Patient in Room 2603

I KNOW YOUR room.
 I lived there for five weeks. I love how you've shoved the bed over against the window, making you much more "one with the outside" and your goal, to get outside of this place.
 I know your pain.
 Yes, this phrase has become comical in its overuse, but in your case, Madame Butterfly, you know I know.
 I am glad we met, you in your robe covered in brightly-winged insects. You call me your mentor, even though I'm your daughter's age. I guess we mentors can be any age, but you also give me strength. It may sound convoluted, but since you are probably smarter than me and you learned English at a much later age, I'll attempt an explanation. By allowing me to feel all-knowing about this stinky disease and by letting me in to help, you are helping me. For the entire summer I've relied on others for help. Now by your simple act of wanting to know more from me, I am able to give a little back. God, it feels good. Thank you, Madame.

So here's a little more "help." I was sitting on my insanely comfortable couch while the rest of my family slept in this Sunday morning and I was thinking about you, sending healing thoughts out from over here in Freedomville. I realize you are in the thick of it right now. You are in that place where the drugs in the bag hanging next to you are really hammering your mind and body. This is "Go Time," M. This is when you rely on everything you've ever known to pull you through.

Remember your own comfy spot at home. Remember your garden and your green thumb. Remember your husband and your daughter, both hovering by your bedside knowing and not knowing what to do. Remember why you signed up to join this planet in the first place. Remember health.

Mostly, remember health. Because it's looking for you and continually asks me about you. It wants so badly to visit and your nurses and doctors are trying to issue it a day pass. I saw it in the ward knocking on other people's doors but it was pounding on yours! Ms. Butterfly, you don't know how badly health feels for you.

But truly, the most important note I can pass on is that very soon you will succumb to health. Even my own five weeks before you, in your room—with that insane cooling vent and the bed that adjusts even when, damn it, you don't want it to adjust—seems to have faded a little from my memory. Only just a little, but a little nevertheless.

And that's the thing. Our cancer is the kind that allows that. Our doctor has never had a failure with this type of blood disease. Life's not over; there's still much more to come. Your eyes tell me you know this and want this. Now let your body realize it. Yes, the medicine that's destroying the cancer is also bringing other sicknesses with it. You can't imagine what was lurking in my intestines a few months ago. But I've seen the way you handle those invaders and I'm impressed.

In some very real ways Madame, you are my mentor. And I am all the better for it.

CHAPTER **35**

# The Kids Are All Right

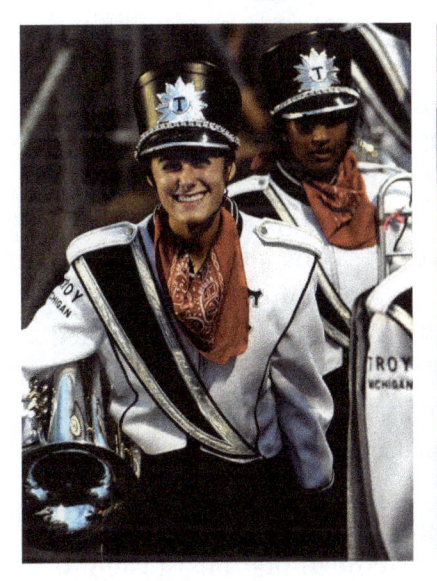

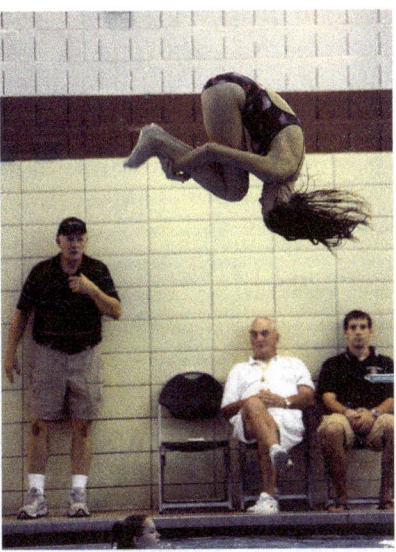

**AFTER A COMBINED** two months in the hospital (three different stays spread out over two different buildings during one summer), one of the things I was looking forward to most was just being a regular ol' dad. Our daughters were forced to fend for themselves during much of their summer break and even if they weren't scraping up road kill and cooking it over a makeshift fire, they were left to their own devices far more than normal.

Pizza, when they weren't fed by an extremely diverse and caring team of friends and family, was on the menu for lunch and dinner more often than not.

But more importantly, with Marci handling all the revenue-generating, the girls had to get themselves places, entertain themselves, take care of stuff they normally wouldn't have to, all the while living in more of a vacuum than ever before. And yet, somehow they thrived. They grew; they expanded their horizons and they reached deep within, finding better versions of themselves (at least that's what I'm telling myself).

Last night's marching band performance (which some people still mistakenly call a football game) and an away diving meet were a great time for us to just be parents, take some snapshots, ooh and ahh over their performances and drive like crazy between high schools because they both happened at roughly the same time. We loved it.

It's the stuff I've taken for granted that gets me. But looking back over my life, I can't say I've ever truly taken the girls for granted. Skye coming out of the womb with a life threatening E. coli bacteria infection and Taylor having to wear a hip/leg brace for the first year of her life tended to make us realize—quite early—how precious life can be. Daddy getting a freak blood disease out of nowhere just magic-marker underlined life's wonder and fragility.

But look at these two last night. Do they look like girls whose infancy was marred by extreme limitations? Listen to them upstairs—first laughing together, now arguing—are they anything but normal, healthy teens? In some very palpable way, they serve as reminders that I can get through *anything* and must get through *everything* in order to remain their proud papa.

There's only one more short interlude where I'll be incarcerated in the health system (for my own good, of course!). And this one's for all the marbles. Then my life, and my family's will continue along the tracks laid out long ago. I hope I'll be the type of survivor who relishes the ordinary and grooves on the everyday. Although in all honesty, and not even with a hint of parental pride, living with these two—and their terrific mother—rarely, if ever, is an ordinary or everyday experience.

CHAPTER **36**

# Far Too Much Time on My Hands

TWIDDLING MY THUMBS, waiting for all the pieces to fall into place for my bone marrow transplant, I start to get antsy. Random thoughts come to mind. Questions begin to plague me. The big questions, you know, things like these:

- What if I didn't invest my money wisely over the years? What if I fell for one of Henry Winkler's Fonzie schemes?
- In "She'll be coming 'round the mountain," who is *she*?
- Did you know the world gullible isn't in the dictionary?
- Why are those primitive cave drawings we've all seen so special? They're crap. My baby nephew could do better and he's never even witnessed an antelope slaughter.
- Would Elvis Costello be more popular if his mom named him after his uncle Abbott?

- Rembrandt used to bilk everyone he ran into. There wasn't a person he didn't try to swindle. He was the original con artist.
- The local synagogue is planning a Passover trip for kids to Seder Pointe.
- Have you ever swum in a carpool? I did once, but got felt up by a Dodge Prowler.
- If one more middle-aged white guy tells me, "you da bomb," I'm just gonna explode.
- I reconnected with my old college friend Christa. She was married for a while to a dude named Stan Ball. She still goes by Christa Ball though since—even though as a little girl it meant nothing—as a grownup, her maiden name, Meth, drew too many late night phone calls.
- Maybe it's me, but I think Trappist monks should have to eat everything they trap.

CHAPTER 37

# Dichotomy

EVERYTHING IS ALL messed up. And in the same breath, everything is perfect.

On the outside, looking in—and honestly, from the inside looking in, too—it appears the misfortunes I've had over the past year have been devastating. Losing my job would be enough to throw me over the edge. Getting another newspaper job and having that paper go out of business after a short few weeks would appear heart-rending. My daughter not getting into the overseas program she dreamed about, or us getting robbed in Paris, both were punches to our familial psyche. Not getting a summer or fall teaching gig after finding my calling as a professor was a blow. Leukemia. Yeah, leukemia. You know the rest.

Sure, each of those losses held gifts for us, hidden in the ruins. But I don't always feel those gifts. I can't honestly sit here and say I'm glad I don't have a job, even though not having one lifts an entire metric ton of weight off my shoulders in terms of needing to get things done, organized, taken care of, worried about.

Some days, like today, I can feel the equal and opposite weight on my shoulders of the cancer. I can feel it dragging at my heels as I sprint for the cure. And the one place where I normally get my solace—the people around me—are some of the ones doing the dragging. Talking to older patients today had the effect of putting the stink eye on my prognosis. Here they were, lined up with their bald heads and face masks—that I too will soon sport—telling me all the things that can go wrong. Each of them having had recurring cancers and at least two marrow transplants. How can you think everything will go smoothly? Do you know you won't be able to cook meals for months? You'll need to have someone around you 24/7. You are susceptible to every disease out there. That hair that's slowly growing back on your head, well, it's about to fall out all over again.

And on and on.

They meant no harm; they just smelled raw meat joining their club and like a freshman initiation, I had to walk the gauntlet. But mixed in with the so-called advice were nuggets I could glean. One guy said he felt like he was back to his normal self right away, even though he wasn't supposed to go out and do things. It was wintertime anyway, so that didn't really bother him. Another person said attitude is everything, which I've often heard. Too bad that claim was immediately dumped on by some of the others there, lined up waiting for their appointments. One of the participants even asked what type of anti-anxiety drug I was on. When I said I was anti-depressant-less, the others chimed in with their pharmacologicals.

It almost made me depressed.

Later, as I was locked into a breathing chamber in an adjacent building, I was thinking about all their jumbled words. The Plexiglas enclosure was supposed to test the many facets of my breathing. For a guy who has a few recent psychological

chapter 37 • 101

issues surrounding not being able to breathe, you don't really want to shut me up in a box with a glorified clothespin over my nose and a large tube protruding from my mouth.

"Now pant quickly ... now inhale ... now exhale, even if it feels like you can't force any more air out," said the technician. The machine actually clogged up and I was supposed to push as hard as I could against the lack of being able to breathe.

Where *were* those anti-anxiety pills?

I realized after my bell jar tests were over that this whole cancer and recovery thing really pisses me off. People telling me their horror stories really pisses me off. Not knowing how long all of this is going to take really pisses me off. Not having any control over it all really pisses me off.

And yet I have the time to write. And yet somehow we are making it work financially. And yet my daughter not being overseas and me not having a job as a professor or photo editor seems to work to our overall advantage right now. I wouldn't wish leukemia or recovery on anyone, but I definitely wouldn't wish it on someone who's busy.

I don't know the cosmic plan. I don't know my own plan. But I'm getting the impression that somehow this is all playing out perfectly, according to some unforeseen diagram.

And yes, that pisses me off too.

CHAPTER **38**

# An Occasional Little Schnuffle

SINCE I PROBABLY bummed you out with my last story, I thought I'd follow up with something useful. One of the biggest raps against me in the working world was I liked to please everybody. I'm so sorry if that displeases you.

But onward and downward.

Friend, do you find yourself snoring at night? Do you wake up wondering why they're working a pneumatic drill in your bedroom? Does your spouse complain? Does this sound like an infomercial?

Well, Dr. Rodney is here to help. One of the benefits of being in the hospital is sharing medical advice with fellow patients, nurses and doctors. After a quick and off-the-cuff conversation with a fellow leukemia patient last month, I found myself wondering about snoring. I actually had to go back, seek her out and ask for clarification because I couldn't believe what I heard.

Deep breathing. It's that simple. She had gone into a sleep clinic months earlier to deal with an apnea issue and one of the main things they taught her was to work on taking deep breaths all throughout the day. Now this part needed clarification.

"Really?" I asked, thinking clarification is best when you only use one word.

"Yes, various times throughout the day, just relax, take several deep breaths through your nose and exhale, if you can, longer than it takes to inhale," she said.

So of course I tried it.

I didn't believe the results. I'm not sure if I believe them yet but something has changed in my sleep patterns; I don't snore nearly as much. My wife was telling me that after my second hospital stay—you know, the one with the blood clot and all—my snoring was downright cacophonic. Sure, it could've been caused by any number of things, but I had been building up to a crescendo for years. Marci even has earplugs resting on her nightstand.

After talking with my fellow patient and doing those deep breathing exercises, apparently my night rumblings have greatly reduced. Remember, this is anecdotal evidence I'm sharing here and you should know never to listen to me. But the deep breathing worked.

Now, several times throughout the day and most every night or before napping—yes, I nap a lot these days—I remember to inhale deeply and exhale even deeper. Sometimes I send a rush of blood to my head, but if I'm lying down, that's not all bad. I have to tell you, I'm surprisingly much more snoreless. (By the way, if you're keeping track of my made-up words, spellcheck doesn't even come close to allowing "snoreless" or "cacophonic." Don't worry, there will certainly be many more.)

While my wife is busy typing at her computer behind me I ask, "So if I were quoting you about my snoring right now, Marci, what would I write?"

"It's not bad at all; an occasional little schnuffle." Apparently I'm not the only one with a creative vocabulary.

I looked it up online and some sites—not the majority by any means, but some sites—list the same exercise. So there you have it. Take this advice or forget about it. Do your best not to yell at me for dispensing quack medicinery if we bump into each other at some future date.

And hey, if you read about anything on the Internet that stops nighttime farting ...

CHAPTER **39**

# A Breath of Fresh Hair

GOD, I LOVE the way the wind feels through my half-inch hair. A big blow has been exhaling through Michigan for many hours now and my tiny follicles, like the long stringy willow tree out back, have been dancing in the breeze.

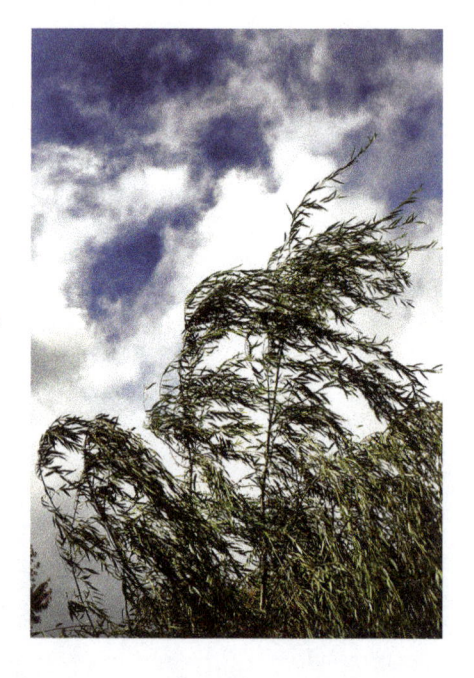

One of the first things they teach you at Cancer College is how your perspective on life will change. I keep waiting for a dramatic shift and all I get are little bitty glimpses of appreciation. The breeze through my hair, which nowadays I "wash" only a few times a week, is one of those moments where I remember to be thankful.

Shampooing used to be a daily drudgery. Wild, unkempt hair in the wind never looked good on me. "Ha," I say to myself now. "Take that, Suave."

You also learn at Leuk U that there are many strange side effects to your treatment. Apparently the tingling in my left arm that I've been feeling for a week and a half isn't a slow-moving heart attack or a stroke taking its time to strike. The technical definition for it is, well, "tingling in the left arm."

A doctor has told me this twice, this week and last. I also heard second-hand from Marci's chiropractor, who strangely knew a whole heap about cancer, that if my tingling was serious, I'd know it by now. I'll leave it up to you to decide which doctor made me feel more assured. (Hint: The first doctor was the one who missed the warning signs for my blood clot).

As I drive home with the windows down and greet Young Man Willow out back, I laugh at how just a few words from a few doctors can completely change my attitude. No longer am I harboring sinister secret enemies slowly springing a trap. Now my biggest fear is psychosomatic illnesses running roughshod in my mind, taunting me with their what-ifs, and their more diabolic "You-should-really-go-to-the-ER-nows."

I love the way my new 'do and the willow tree just let the wind blow without a care. Neither are re-shaped, even temporarily, nor do they seem to stress out that there's a breeze. A logical leap would be for me to wish that for myself, but I think not caring or not being affected just aren't in my tool kit. I am affected by lots of things, everything. My greatest strength is my greatest weakness. Its name is sensitivity.

I'll probably still worry, just a little, that the tingling is a harbinger of something nefarious. I'll wonder why I need to collect 24 hours-worth of urine in a bright red jug before checking in for my stem cell swap, my bone marrow transplant. And when the centimeter or two of hair falls out, then grows back, I'll probably once again care how I look after a stiff breeze or showerless morning. My perspective will shift. But will my vanity?

CHAPTER **40**

# Born Again?

DOWN IN DETROIT, at my new home away from home, the Karmanos Cancer Institute (*http://bit.ly/VN2Swd*), people have wonderful words for their services. The person who walks me or pushes me from one appointment to the next is called my "Navigator." The woman who plays the role of nurse, contact person and barrier-buster is my "Coordinator." But my favorite word is "Rebirth." My coordinator, Stacey, used that word yesterday to describe the simply miraculous process that begins on Friday, October 8th.

By getting my brother's stem cells, I will be like a newborn, she told me. It brought tears to my eyes when she reiterated that they're not playing around. This is all about a cure, not just remission. She made her case even stronger when she reminded me I'd need my newborn baby shots all over again by the time I'm one year old.

Honestly.

My diphtheria, tetanus, measles and all the other shots I got back in the Stone Age are no longer valid. (Yes, I'll get them again and no, I'm not worried about suddenly turning into a stump or whatever the anti-inoculation crowd fears these days.)

The epic coincidence—that I was originally born right there, in the same medical complex 47 years ago—has left my metaphoric jaw dragging on the proverbial pavement.

Back then, as the family fable goes, Mom and Dad swung in for a milkshake on the way to the hospital. I was their third kid and I think maybe Pop was being a bit cavalier. I blame my insane appetite for coffee milkshakes on this prenatal pit stop.

To be honest, I kind of like the thought of being a newborn. It allows me to reconfigure my life based on a very real biologic restructuring. If I have to attend elementary school again, I know I'll breeze right through. In college maybe I'll study to become a Wall Street banker instead of an unemployed journalist. I can't wait for my lucrative bonus package just for being potty trained.

Babies don't have to face the worries like I encountered recently while talking with the diabolic Humana or Aetna insurance cartels. They told me curtly over the phone that they simply won't insure me or my family. Insurance corporations were formed to help people. Now, apparently, they *are* people. I hope they don't get mugged in some dark alley.

But most importantly, this process helps me put old patterns to bed and gives me the chance to rally around the rebirth and adopt new processes. This, of course, will probably turn out to be total bullshit. But at least now, on this side of the procedure, I can pretend I'll change dramatically.

The biggest change I'm hoping for, as a baby just learning about computers, is that I won't have a pathologic fear about emptying my trash because I could've inadvertently put something important in there.

Maybe I'll finally choose Canon over Nikon, or boxers over briefs.

And if I'm lucky, I can bring my daily fear level down from Red to maybe Blue. My fears aren't the overt "Taliban-raping-my-dog" kind of fears. I tend to fear the inane stuff, like uttering the wrong thing in a social situation or making someone mad for something silly I said.

But for the real authority on what I should do differently I ask, pivoting my ripped up desk chair, "Taylor, pretend I'm being reborn. What should I do differently this time around?"

"Take risks, Daddy," my daughter says.

Oh cool, I'm going to become an adventurer, maybe jump out of airplanes or get over my scubaphobia and search for sunken ships. I try for more clarification but she's back to texting as she walks out the door to driver's training.

There's more in that statement, I know. And when I'm a little baby goo-gooing around the place we'll get to the soul of it, I'm sure.

I hope when I'm a baby again I just eat, poop and love. To live in oneness with the universe would be fabulous. I know other stuff will crowd in and I stand absolutely no chance of remaining so enlightened, though. Heck, even the Dalai Lama has a Twitter account (*http://bit.ly/TV33pJ*). Hopefully I'll learn the most important lesson and not take myself as seriously as I do. But I realize that even planning for a near future where I don't take myself too seriously is already, in itself, taking myself too seriously.

And just like that, the mind games also experience their own rebirth.

CHAPTER 41

# Tenth Floor

I THOUGHT THE guy down the hall was making fun of me. On one of the ubiquitous dry erase boards posted on the 10th floor of the Karmanos Cancer Institute, there was a guy's name, Ray, spelled with a giant outlandish R.

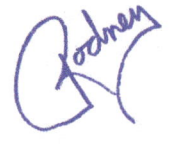

"Wait, that's my R," I thought to myself, "someone's already messing with me; this is cool." Tracking him down on one of the many laps we're all supposed to walk, (your boy Rodney's aiming for two miles a day; in your face, office-dwellers!), I found out he signs his name with the same insane R. Better yet, he does the same with his last name, which also begins with an R. I can't share it with you since I think I'm already in trouble with HIPA.

Other than the signature and the cool view of Motor City Casino's (*http://aol.it/TV3514*) lights at night combined with the Ambassador Bridge (*http://bit.ly/TV3515*), there's not a lot of surprising stuff going on here. And that's fine by me. Well, there *is* that frosted glass in my door that, when you flip a light switch, changes to clear. That's pretty surprising. But for the most part, I am doing what I've done during previous hospital stays: read, imbibe chemo, do laps, get bored, mess with the nurses, eat, sleep when I can, mess with the nurses some more, repeat cycle.

I keep feeling like there's something more I should be doing. I guess the beautiful fall weekend we've had doesn't hurt as much knowing that the leaves will be handled by someone else. (Daughters, I'm talking to you.)

But my job and pastime these days is health. That pretzel I'm about to eat, does it contribute overall to my well-being? I jolly well hope so. But profoundly more importantly; why can't I take a good, righteous dump these days? Is my family right and I'm literally anal retentive?

Little by little, my fears of another blood clot slip away. The waning cold that's been waning for a few weeks now also seems to be—hmmm, how do I put this?—waning. The side benefit to being cooped up all night and day here is the knowledge that a medical professional is only steps away. I've never been a hypochondriac, but this stupid cancer has caused me to pay more attention to the clues skulking around my body. And just as I surveyed the brilliance of that last sentence, they called a Code Blue over the loudspeaker and my sphincter clenched. "It's another part of the hospital. It's another disease. It's another 'nother other," I assure myself.

Focus on the fun. Remind myself of the positive. Yeah, I had a deadly disease, but I got an iPad out of the deal. Sure, these bags are pumping poisons into my system, but didn't I enjoy all those cheeseburgers and pizzas over the last month and a half? Okay, there may be someone coding on another floor, but I can't control that.

And, as if on cue from the great standup comedian in the sky, my wonderful nurse Melissa walks in to explain how my shots will be handled. "We poke you in the evening then put you to bed," she says.

"You don't know what that sounds like," I reply.

"Yes, I do; you may need a cigarette afterward."

Messing with the nurses means they can mess right back.

CHAPTER **42**

# A Transplant Tutorial

## What to Expect When You're Expectorating

SINCE MY GOAL in life is to teach people about complicated medical procedures, here's a quick primer on stem cell transplants or the bone marrow process. Here's your pal, Dr. Rodney, back to explain it all. Stem cell or bone marrow; they seem to be used interchangeably these days. At no point in the upcoming procedure is any of my brother's marrow extracted from his bones.

Here is what's going to happen as I approach my new birthday on Friday. My body is being wracked with lots of different chemicals in order to pound my forces into submission. Use any war analogy you wish. The most important thing they're going for is the stuff that produces my blood, my bone marrow. Other transplants are different, obviously. If you're in for a kidney transplant they handle things differently. The same is true for a full cranial transplant. Probably for hair plug transplants as well.

My marrow and blood is healthy right now; it's in remission. But there's a chance the leukemia could come back.

That's what this is all about. We want to dramatically reduce the chance anything will come back. That's why they call it "The Cure."

Okay, so what actually happens? While they've been bombarding me, they've been doing the opposite to my brother Scott. They are giving him injections of Neupogen, which increases his production of white blood cells. Each day this week he has to take the thousand-dollar-a-day syringe and give himself a shot. No one looks forward to Neupogen—in some people it makes your bones feel like they're exploding from within. Hopefully he won't pull the plug on this project due to pain. There are some fabulous pain medications that work. Sorry, Scott, I don't think this qualifies you for medical marijuana just yet; you'll have to get yours the old-fashioned way.

This Friday, he will report to duty on the 10th floor, just a few steps away from my room. They'll start an IV going in one of his arms, thread the tube through a machine and pump the blood back into his other arm. But that machine in the middle will be extracting his stem cells, which are the worker bees who want to create good, solid, warm blood.

It will take about four hours for this to unfold and when it's complete, he's free to go home. They then take that bag and bring it to me, hot and steamy, and just hang it up on my IV pole and slurp, slurp, slurp like a baby vampire I go.

Since we carry the exact same 10 out of 10 genetic markers that they look for, our genes are a perfect match. But that doesn't mean his cells won't reject me. Yeah, that's weird; in this procedure, the new body of cells can reject the older, established cells there. It's called Graft vs. Host Disease and you supposedly want a little bit of brotherly squabbling, but not a full out Hatfields vs. McCoys.

This potential battle will be omnipresent for months, or even years. In the meantime, post stem cell transfer, I'll need to be very germophobic and avoid crowds. I can't even do some normal things like cook my own food or go outside without a mask. That's the future. Right now, I just need to concentrate on dealing with my body as it prepares for my brother's precious gift of life.

I hope that clears things up.

CHAPTER **43**

# My Main Marrow Man

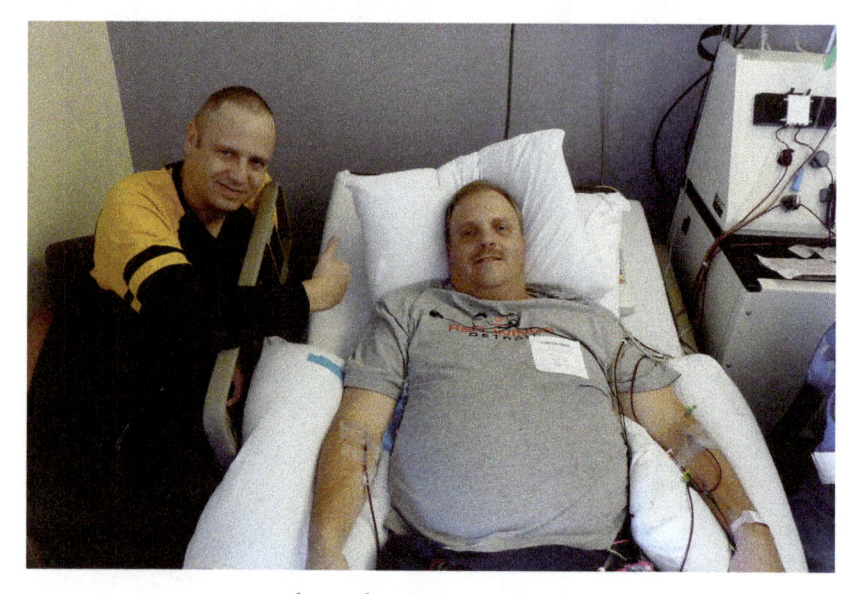

photo by Joanne Curtis

M**Y BROTHER PHONED** me this morning and asked, "So, how's it feel to have me inside of you?"

And with that, we were back to our idiot brotherly ways. No more of this "Thanks for saving my life," or "You know I'd do anything for ya, man." It felt good. Although, he ended the call with "I love you," and I replied "Thanks blood, love ya too."

It adds a funny, weird dynamic to a relationship when one of the participants gives such a tremendous gift. My mom buying him and his wife a new bed doesn't come close to evening out the score. No, I'm not looking around for an opportunity to return the favor, but maybe our next round of golf is on me (note: I said *maybe*, Scott).

I've never loved the thought of being in someone's debt and have always paid off my bills on time. This is one of those things that can never be paid off, unless I somehow arrange to have him trapped on top of a burning building and I learn how to fly a helicopter. Knowing Scott and his firefighting skills, he'd refuse the flight, find an emergency exit and save a bunch of orphans on the way down.

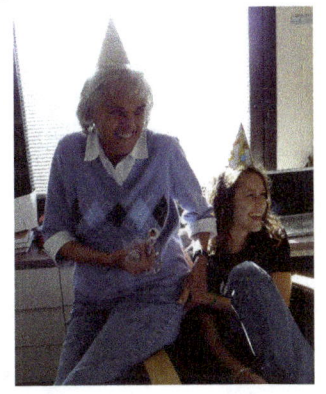

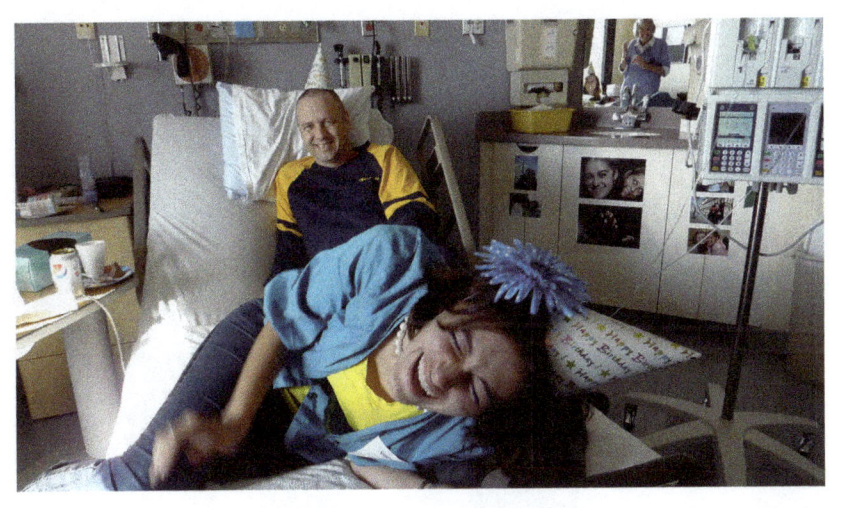

**photo by Marci Curtis**

His smart-ass remark this morning helped alleviate some of my silly repay-the-debt thinking. I can go back to luxuriating in my second Wendy's (*http://www.wendys.com/*) cheeseburger transfusion since Stem Cell Friday, (which is one infusion more than my Buddy's Pizza (*http://bit.ly/VN2SMC*) intake). If this is

chapter 43 • 119

what it's like to have my brother's marrow, I'm lovin' it. Wait, that's a McDonald's theme … Ohhhhh, iced coffee ... Yummm.

Seriously though, this weekend has been wonderful. I feel like a new man (*insert joke here*), and even though I know the effects of my final round of chemo haven't fully hit me, I can still see an ever-growing light at the end of this Tunnel of Love freak show.

"Life," as a few of my cool shirts here say, "is good." Even Detroit looks beautiful outside my window as the pockets of trees all around us start showing off. And this is where I know I'm in some sort of weird reverie—even the people a few streets over, along the formerly notorious Cass Corridor look happy to be outside enjoying the sunshine.

Man, who knew a couple cheeseburgers and some bone marrow would be so good for the soul?

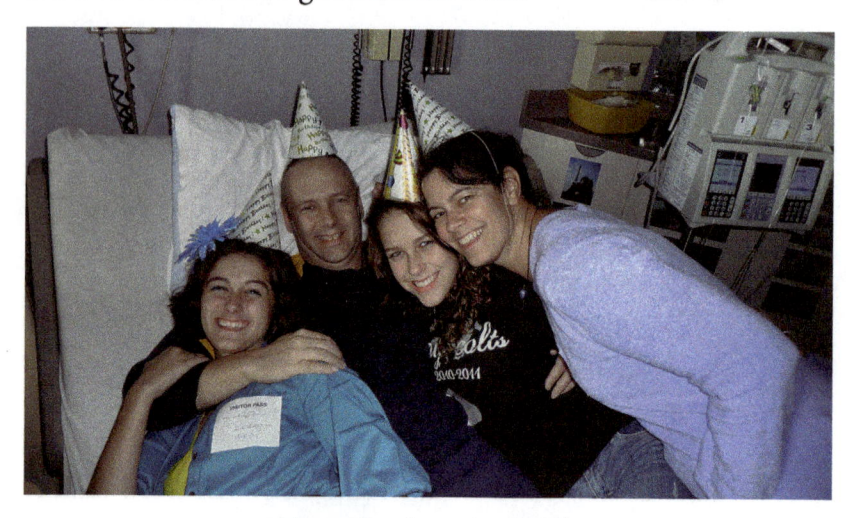

**photo by Joanne Curtis**

CHAPTER **44**

# Nadir and Me

I KEEP GETTING emails from Nadir. So far I haven't hit REPLY yet. Now Nadir has taken to calling me and leaving long, soothing voicemail messages. He's done this three times before and each time he's been right. But this time I just haven't felt like playing his game.

Nadir isn't some slick foreign spy or a wealthy aristocrat you'd find at the Baccarat tables. Nadir is the time period after chemotherapy where all my blood counts are at their lowest. The chemicals slowly bring my body down to a point where I am sluggish, sick-like, feel as though the flu would be a better option and generally would really just rather stare at the ceiling.

But Nadir is important. Because now my brother's stem cells can have the run of the place. Come on in, my body says, bring that ham sandwich with you and by all means make yourself at home. After all, there's nothing in my system stopping him.

After the three previous Nadirs I popped out on the other side feeling oh so much better. One thing my pesky former doctor told me on the day he diagnosed me was, "You'll probably feel better after all this is over." I couldn't really believe that, but each time I've recovered from the chemo, my blood counts indicate I'm much better than a baseline test I had last year before getting laid off.

And that's where I'm sitting now. Only this time there's no more Nadirs afterward. There's no more chemo. There's never been a time in my life where I've looked forward to being sick. But too, there's never been a time when I've been sick on purpose and have known things on the other side will be brilliant.

So I'm about to pick up the phone and talk to my slick buddy on the other end. I imagine he's stroking his goatee, sipping some fabulous drink and smiling with a wicked yet playful gleam. I'm where I should be and the last four doctors and nurses who visited me left my room laughing.

Deal the cards Nadir. And hand me one of those fabulous drinks.

CHAPTER 45

# It's not My-in, It Must be Urine

THEY MONITOR MY urine here. The total cost of my stay to the insurance company will probably be about $250,000, but to the people that have to dump my collected urine, that cost is far too low. The nurses down here at Karmanos need to know how much my output is keeping pace with my input, so no toilet for me; it's a series of random jugs, some of them placed bedside in the middle of the night, some elsewhere. I'm the Easter Bunny of pee.

The nurses find my hidden treasures, measure them, then dump them. There's a special spot—or pot—in Valhalla, for the ones that have to do it most often.

Amazing Nurse Melissa was attending to my daily medications and IV drips when she stepped into the bathroom only to find a few empty jugs. "Hmmm," she thought. "Has Rodney slowed down his output?" And here's what she asked . . . wait for it . . .

*"Did somebody dump urine on you today?"*

Never let it be said that I'm *not* an opportunist. I know sometimes I make inappropriate jokes or laugh in the face of cancer. A "golden" opportunity like that just screams for a comeback. But I whiffed. I think my response was, "Oh, I didn't realize we were in one of those relationships, you and I."

Yeah, lame. But you have to give me one or two style points for hearing the double entendre. She immediately exploded with laughter. So did her nurse helper. I'm the first to laugh at my own jokes, so I was actually clutching my infected belly. It hurt to laugh like that.

"And there we have it," Melissa said. "We've now degraded our professional medical relationship to the point of golden showers."

Is laughter the best medicine? For me it is. So much of cancer recovery, and indeed *any* type of healing is how you look at it. I've been told by doctors, nurses and former patients that attitude counts for everything, when it comes to the difference between success and failure. That's an enormous wake up call. If attitude is everything, why in the name of everything would I be negative or grumpy or pessimistic or glum?

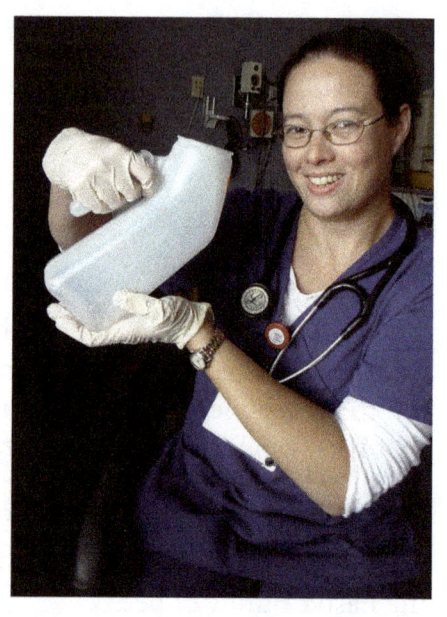

Oh, I know why, because it's freaking **cancer** we're talking about here and cancer is by its very definition negative. You don't hear people talking about a gorgeous sunset or a fantastic meal by saying, "Man, that baked ziti was so creamy and delicious, it's downright *cancerous*."

I'm not trying to tell you that all it takes is to smile and ignore the scary stuff. Nor am I saying people who succumb to the disease somehow failed. Definitely not; far from it. What I am saying, is nurses, medical professionals and even the cleaning folks can tell, when someone checks into a ward, which patient is most likely to whip the disease and which one is likely to have a significantly more difficult time.

I've spewed a lot of crazy stuff since I was diagnosed. And let's face it, I was even crazier beforehand. But the one takeaway I've gleaned is to simply push the positive.

It's like calisthenics sometimes, making yourself cross over to the sunny side of the street. But studies have actually shown how new neuron pathways get re-routed by thinking about something differently. If your response to a boss, an illness, your in-laws or even the Kardashians is a continual, predictable, negative path, then simply thinking differently about them can re-wire your brain.

That's some heady stuff (literally). Thinking makes it so? Attitude is everything? When the people around me say much of healing is mental, it almost sounds like magical thinking. But I'll try anything, so I force the desperation out of my disposition.

But then, nighttime shows up.

Along with nighttime, arrives an insane gut disease which is so contagious, visitors have to wear paper gowns and rubber gloves when they enter my room.

Night also brings Neupogen, shots which explode my bones so the stem cells can settle into my body and bring along their furniture, a couple friends and even a cardboard box or two of old eight-track tapes they couldn't eBay.

And finally, mucositis sneaks on in. It's a mouth and throat disease so painful, it feels like I sleepwalked down to a Rouge River foundry, grabbed a Dixie cup full of molten steel and swallowed it on a bar bet.

Through this all, do I remain positive and upbeat? No, man, *heck no*! Remember the part about the exploding bones? No, this is beyond pain. But as I reach over and grab the weird device that sucks spit out of my mouth, I realize this too shall pass. It's only for now. And that's the key. It will all be over, eventually.

Of that, I *am* positive.

CHAPTER 46

# I Hear a Symphony

I AM HOME. I am recovering. I am richer for the experience.

And I'm not speaking in metaphors here. I am actually richer than I was before I entered Karmanos. Thanks to the amazing generosity of the Detroit journalism community and the far-flung print purchasers (from New York to Hawaii) who decided now was the time to pick up a print, my soon-to-be canceled insurance coverage just became a little less fearful.

My buddies and former colleagues at the *Detroit News* and *Free Press*—on my behalf—sold a great selection of history's most memorable photographs from their archives, all to benefit my family. Also, many area photographers added their favorites to the gallery for purchase.

The names behind the scenes are endless. In fact, it took some journalistic digging on my part just to find out who to begin privately thanking.

The photos were brilliant and whether it was The Supremes and Berry Gordy or a 1920s rum runner, I can't adequately say how blown away I am to be the recipient of the sale of such quietly earth-shaking moments in Detroit's history.

You've felt me bash you over the head with this before, but the connections you make throughout the years with people—even those that you thought were just casual work acquaintances—are always a part of you and should never be taken lightly.

As our COBRA wanes and we consider self-employment insurance, long term disability, Blue Cross and other possibilities, it makes it less scary to be adrift with so many friends paddling our lifeboat.

And way up there in our makeshift crow's nest, I think I just heard someone yell **"Land, ho!"**

CHAPTER **47**

# Our Hallucination

I WAS SITTING with my cousin-buddy Chris in the parking lot outside my daughter Skye's play, waiting for the crowd to finish entering the auditorium so I could ghost in and sit in the back, wearing a germ-free mask. I told him the following story and he said I should share it. I feel very weird about doing so, for reasons you're about to find out.

There were a few nights back in the hospital that I was on heroin or opium and I really can't remember what happened. That sounds like the beginning to a really great college story, but unfortunately this one involves poo. The actual drug I was imbibing, every 15 minutes via a convenient pump mechanism, was Dilaudid—a derivative of morphine. "Deluded" is a better name for the painkiller.

Not going into too much gross detail about my gross motor skills, let's just take it as assumed that eating and swallowing were out and pooping was in—way in. There's one night in particular that I have not been able to get independent verification on, but a shadowy part of my memory recalls being hoisted into rubber pants and being told to just sit there while a battalion of midnight shift workers took care of "things." I know I wasn't imagining this.

But I probably was.

The doctor told me one of Dilaudid's side effects was hallucinations. I told him, seriously as I could, "I'm not having any problems with that until I close my eyes and the room fills with people I've never met."

One of the greatest benefits about being a jokester is people think you're kidding when you're really being serious, but shouldn't be. I wasn't ready for the drug to go bye-bye. Neither were all my friends, who instantly arrived whenever my eyelids blinked. They were a great group of partiers who would hang out everywhere in the place, gravity not being a concern to them. Were they the dead? Were they from another realm? Were they Fig Newtons of my imagination?

None of them were evil, many didn't even seem to notice me and only a few would sit or float bedside and carry on a brief conversation. No, I can't remember what they had to say, but there was a whole passel of them just enjoying the jam of being in my head and showing me an alternate reality.

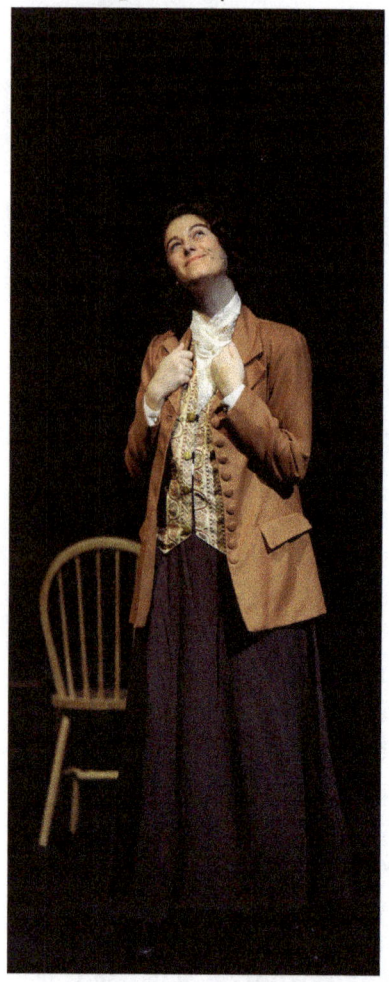

**photo by Marci Curtis**

130 • A "Cute" Leukemia

I should've done more drugs in college.

Having beings and buddies, not-too-real but nevertheless present, was a pleasant surprise. I wasn't prepared to call them hallucinations but I wasn't ready to dismiss them entirely. As I tap this out—munching on magnesium-producing brown rice with a nightcap of yogurt to continue curing my insides—I look at the hallucinations as wacky windows into something else. Whether they were real or imagined, I'm glad for their existence. They were nonchalant and I felt comfortable around them. That may be the best message ever.

If that's what other realms are about, I can handle it. If that's where my mind goes in the end, I can handle that too. It's these glimpses that I've gotten along the way that provide a sense of something eternal.

And then as if scripted, my cousin and I float into the auditorium and there's my daughter on stage talking in "Our Town" about how dead people finally understand there's something eternal to all of this. Here's what she, I mean Thornton Wilder, said:

> We all know that something is eternal, and it ain't houses, and it ain't names, and it ain't the Earth and it ain't even the stars … everybody knows in their bones that something is eternal, and that something has to do with human beings. All the greatest people ever lived have been telling us that for 5,000 years and yet you'd be surprised how people are always losing hold of it. There's something way down deep that's eternal about every human being.

In the handout program, she dedicated this next line to her mom and me:

> Do any human beings ever realize life while they live it? The saints and poets, maybe—they do some.

If my daughter sees Marci and me as a saint and a poet, we've already achieved eternity. And that's not being deluded one bit.

CHAPTER **48**

# The Beginning of the NDE

FOOD ARRIVES AT our place on an almost routine basis these days. Organized by some incredible friends, a chuck wagon rolls up to our house several times a week in the form of our kids' friends' parents (if I'm allowed to use double apostrophes). The meals have been luscious and much appreciated. And wow, the stories that have arrived, steaming hot, have also been delicious.

Yesterday, I had the pleasure of meeting one of the parents whom I'd never run into before. Her story was phenomenal. Having had brain surgery after brain surgery over the years, the woman could more than empathize with my plight. But when she told me she actually clinically died twice, I knew I had to ask.

"Did you see the tunnel?" I almost rudely inquired. To which she simply responded, with a large smile, "Oh, yes."

To elaborate: for years I've been interested in Near Death Experiences (NDE). I've read widely about different people's and different culture's experiences with them and to say I'm intrigued by the phenomenon is a gross understatement. I've only actually met a handful of people who have agreed to talk to me personally about them. So when I see an opportunity, I swoop in all vulture-like.

Her story was routine and earth-shaking. A huge percentage of these experiences follow her narrative, but when it happens to you it's anything but mundane. What I'm told is that she was at a routine dentist appointment—nothing to do with all her brain tumor work—when she somehow got penicillin, which she is allergic to. She ended up dead on the floor.

A great white light tunnel hovered in front of her and she described a profound feeling of happiness, joy and ultimate, unconditional love. "Once you go there, believe me, you never look back," she explained.

Being nosy (otherwise known as being a journalist) I pushed even further. "Who did you see?" Everyone reports seeing somebody or some being. "Oh, my grandma showed up and that's why I'm here today. She told me I had too many commitments to my small children and husband and to leave them now wouldn't be right at all. So I came back."

She then described coming to in the ambulance and being discombobulated but remembering the soul-releasing experience of pure love. God, do I love hearing people talk like that. She went on to say the little things here on Earth are just that, little, minor details that shouldn't be given too much weight.

She gave me directions on heating up the wonderful dinner, told me she absolutely adored my daughters, then floored me by asking for a hug before departing. "Heavens, yes," I thought joyfully, otherworldly, gratefully, "I'll take a hug."

So when my ladies arrived home, I showed the food off and shared the story. My wife quickly pointed out, "Oh, it sounds a lot like Grandma."

Taylor agreed, but I had somehow forgotten the story. It turns out Marci's grandma had a very similar experience after the unsuccessful C-section of her first child. Way back in the 1930s, she temporarily died and so did her baby. As she was hovering in that place between life and death she saw her husband bent over, weeping uncontrollably. But here's the thing; she also saw the overwhelmingly beautiful light and was drawn to it, like all souls would be. But no, she stopped somehow and realized that both her child's death and her own death would be too much for her husband to bear. So she went back.

For years, she told that story to the next four children she successfully birthed and to some of her grandkids as well. She always told my wife she didn't fear death and actually was kind of looking forward to it. Living to a ripe old age of 93, she apologized to Marci before going into surgery on my wife's birthday. "I'm sorry, I don't want to mar your birthday with my death," she told Marci.

Obviously she knew something, because she let go on that very day. But I don't think anybody in the extended family felt an overwhelming mourning, because of everything she'd told them all her life.

There's comfort in food and found awakenings. I don't know whether everyone would agree, but I imagine people who've had these sagas look at their metaphysical experiences as silver linings amidst their own personal tragedies.

To us, outsiders who've never had the fortune or misfortune of experiencing such trauma, their stories are gifts far more impressive than Blu-ray players, iPhones or new cars. Their gifts are guideposts along our own epic sagas and there's nothing like pausing during our journey and seeing light at the end of the tunnel. Or as my childhood friend Marc wrote recently, "There's cake at the end of that funnel."

CHAPTER 49

# You Asked About the Meaning of Life

Dear _____,

When we finished talking the other day, I couldn't help but feel I left you hanging. You've been my friend for many, many years and even though I couldn't completely explain what it all means, I felt as though I just gave you some pat, standard answers. I apologize for that.

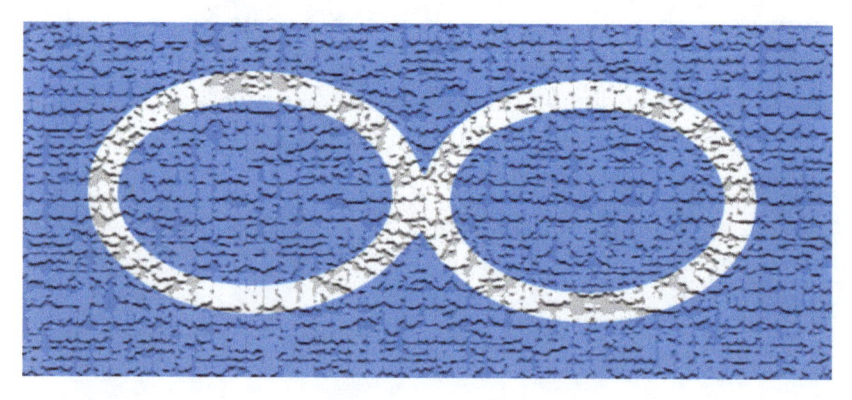

But it's a tough question, "What's the meaning of life?" You and I have known for years that there's more to our saga than is apparent in everyday, 9–5 life. We've spoken many times about there being invisibles, intangibles that help us or benevolently exist as buffers or soft bumpers gently bouncing us in more or less the proper direction if we are sensitive enough to feel them.

And you, with your Protestant upbringing, have long felt the tug of higher planes and beings who, even though you were indoctrinated more than most, still hold a tender place in your soul. So really, your question doesn't ask if there's a greater construct or wider plan, but more, what do we do with this information once it's firmly taken hold in our gut.

I hear you. I think billions of humans hear you too. They've heard your question since conscious thought was a part of primitive humanity. It has plagued civilization throughout the millenniums and yes, I used the word "plague." In some aspects, it gets in our way and causes undue stress. But in other ways, it forces us to ask why we bother getting up in the morning.

I am by no means a sage, advisor or guidance counselor. Nor did my run-in with leukemia bring out a mystical, magical essence, no matter how badly I wished it would have. I'm just another guy with a keyboard trying to explain things through my own warped perspective. But maybe, just maybe, my viewpoint makes sense to you.

I think we're here, as my favorite author Richard Bach (*http://richardbach.com/*) writes, to learn and to love. But we're also here to experience, form inter-tangled relationships, get dirty and messy and deal with issues that we haven't fully dealt with in this or previous lifetimes.

Yes, I'm one of those odd ducks who feels our souls have been around forever and have visited this and other realms again and again. It seems to me that when we jump off this plane, we rest up for a while in the afterworld, have some amazing ambrosia, catch up with our pen pals then decide to do it all over again only this time as pygmies or dolphins or pretzel thieves.

But why? Why experience life? How the heck should I know? But I do know this: the very fact that you and I communicated a few days ago and the very fact that we've been friends for so long is part of the answer. We are sharing this acid trip along with zillions of others past, present and future. So you have to find stuff along the way that juices you and makes the struggle worthwhile and fun.

You've done that. You have your family and your travels and your seeking. So maybe if you're looking for an answer, flip it around and look at the question. Why are we doing this? Maybe partly it's to ask why we're doing this. See my point? By simply asking the question you have received your answer.

Tricky, eh?

If that doesn't help; if finding the answer in amongst the question is too trite for you, I apologize. I've given you the learning/loving/connection spiel. So the only other thing I can try is to share where I've struck gold.

I've found meaning in sharing my life with others. I've found meaning through my family. I've found meaning through travel. I've found meaning through the visual arts. I've found meaning through yanking words out of nowhere and tapping them into submission. I've found meaning through teaching. I've found meaning through the love of friends. I've found meaning through deep, intimate love. I've found meaning through deep, intimate food. I've found meaning through humor. I've found lint in my pockets.

That's about the best I can do and I should've told you all this earlier. But that's the thing about conversations; they can last a lifetime.

CHAPTER 50

# Yoga, the Ultimate Sin

I ENJOYED MY morning, parked in front of the television and sinning like a man destined for the abyss, while I slowly breathed deeply and stretched my aching muscles. I was practicing yoga, attempting to coax my body back into some semblance of normalcy. While doing so, I was apparently committing a mortal sin against Christianity.

Those are some steep consequences for using the Nintendo Wii.

It caught my attention the other day when a casual chat with a number of college friends on Facebook turned heated as we discussed how the ancient practice of yoga puts your soul in jeopardy. If you're a Christian in good standing, who treats people decently, you can suddenly be a candidate for the fiery depths if you so much as breathe deeply or sit in any way remotely resembling a lotus flower.

In response to a Hindu group trying to acquaint Westerners with its roots, *The New York Times* reported that the president of the Southern Baptist Theological Seminary said the practice imperiled the souls of Christians who engage in it.

All this time I thought it just imperiled my ability to hold back gas while doing funny body twists. If you've never tried yoga, it's one of the best ways to unfortunately elicit a fart amongst a group of leotarded women bending in silence.

Now I have to worry about going to a hell that I don't even believe in.

The fight between Hindus and Christians over the topic of who owns yoga is about as absurd as arguing over a fantasy soccer or cricket league (Yes—those, unlike hell, exist). Can't people just go to their community center in peace, roll out some mats and do dopey-looking things for an hour? (Note: This is the reason why I do it at home now, in front of the Wii; I look terribly silly, but don't have to worry about the escaped eruptions delineated earlier).

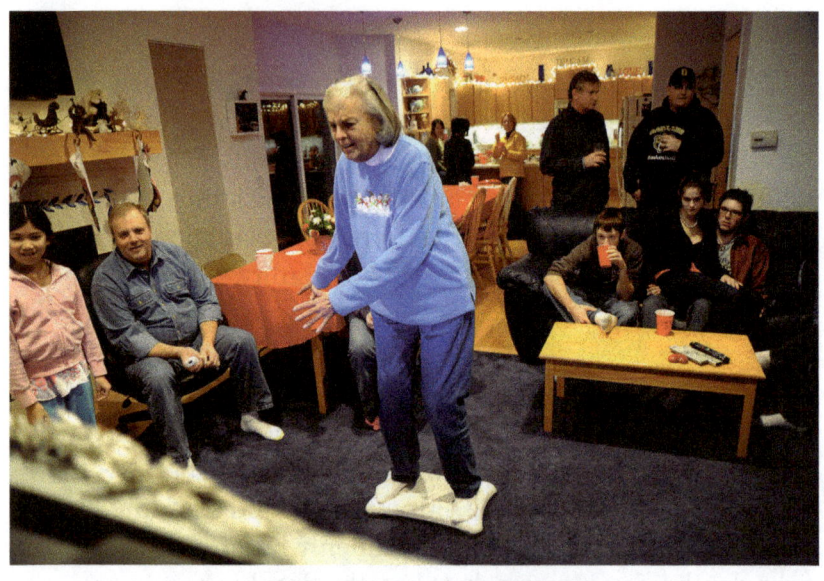

**Even my dear Christian mother is now going to hell, just for a Wii bit.**

At the end of every session we say to each other "*Namaste*." It means, in totally heretical laymen's terms, "The light in me

140 • A "Cute" Leukemia

honors and bows to the light in you." Who can find fault in that? Who cares whether it began in the mystical east eons ago or the phantasmic '60s of Berkeley, California?

And while we're at it, who cares what other people do to relax, de-stress, exercise or build muscle tone as long as it's not illegal and doesn't harm small woodland creatures? When I mentioned to my collegiate associates on Facebook that God has many different names, one person I hadn't even thought about for 25 years told me how wrong I was.

I didn't know I was being so ignorant thinking we were all talking about basically the same thing. But then again, I didn't have my Nintendo console there to help me. And besides, my daughter had the *Super Monkey Ball* disk in the Wii's drive. Once you start taking spiritual advice from a monkey hopped up on Red Bull you know things are getting a little bananas.

Namaste.

CHAPTER 51

# The Worst Christmas Card Ever

"Thankfully Daddy didn't go to heaven. We wish you a happy 2011!"

Thus ended the most inappropriate and raunchy Christmas greeting we've ever conceived.

Here's the background. Imagine two funny teens sitting around in pajamas on a Saturday afternoon, a mom who has her first free weekend in months and a facetious father. The living room was like the mythic backstage writer's room for any given

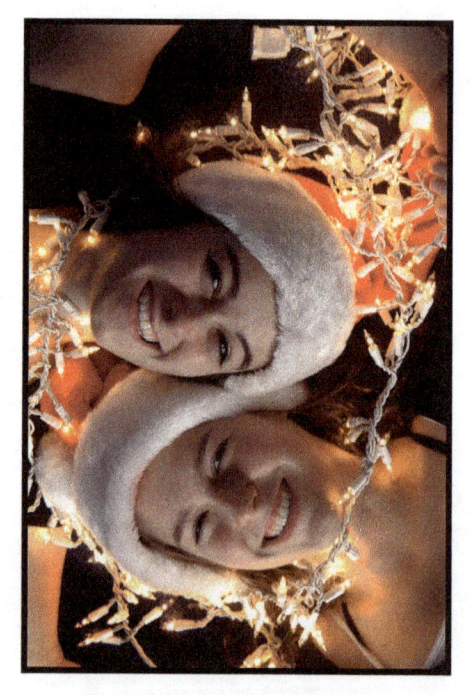

photo by Marci Curtis

comedy show and no holds were barred, although they really should've been.

Our mission was to complete the Curtis Christmas card and get it off to the printer. No one was allowed to go anywhere until we had it down. The obvious problem was how to publicly share what a rough year we had. In the end we went with accentuating the positive while not ignoring the negative. That was in the end though.

Leading up to it, we were laughing our butts off. It seemed that each one of us pushed the other to say something even nastier, as long as it rhymed. Jokes flew back and forth about getting robbed in France, rear-ended in Troy and cancer of the blood among other things.

It was cathartic as hell.

My wonderful daughters and amazing wife sat there shaking with laughter, tears rolling down their cheeks. Pain and sadness can bring people together, but laughing about it also has an incredible curative power. None of us have had that type of prolonged, insane howling in, I don't know how long.

Hilarity helped heal.

Eventually nixing the idea of printing out the X-rated version of our card, we decided instead to just keep that one to ourselves. The regular card is cute, fun and far more holiday-appropriate.

CHAPTER **52**

# Honest Officer, It's the Ambien!

TO HELP ME sleep through some of these long winter's naps, the doctor has prescribed me a bit of Ambien (*http://bit.ly/TV35hq*). Imagine my delight when I read the following on the enclosed instructions (and in the words of Dave Barry, "I'm not making this up"):

*After taking Ambien, you may get up out of bed while not being fully awake and do an activity that you do not know you are doing. The next morning, you may not remember that you did anything during the night. Activities include: driving a car, eating food, talking on the phone, having sex, etc.*

So if you've seen me late at night cruising the seedier parts of Troy and Birmingham with a falafel in one hand and cell phone in the other as I look for hookers (*http://bit.ly/TV35hs*), just realize it's not me. It's the Ambien. I can show you my doctor's note if need be.

Come to think of it, right now it's 1:18 in the morning. I hope I remember this tomorrow. Oh yeah, I totally will; it's written with strawberry jam on a large Pizzapapalis (*http://bit.ly/TV35hv*).

And an enormous wombat is editing it for me as we speak.

CHAPTER 53

# You Are My Person of the Year

You MAKE ME laugh, or laugh nervously along with me as I say something vastly inappropriate. You look past my laughter, see the deeper and still decide to smile. You fart at just the right moment.

You knew I needed something to hold onto the second the news came from that stupid doctor. You saw your world come crashing down, but you took those cement-filled steps over to me as I stared into the abyss.

You gained weight just to be in communion with me as you fed my dwindling body. You heard me late at night when I didn't even know I was calling. You worked all day, took care of our family and still visited me.

You believed all along that this was curable, beatable, smashable. You've been right all along. You are my press secretary and wing-woman, fielding calls and questions from everywhere. You never, never, never let me forget I'm a man.

You tell me my skin stretches beautifully over an excellently-shaped scalp. You support us economically, socially and psychically. You are my favorite favorite. You put up with the weird and bizarre as I emerge from the shadow.

You are a tremendous financial planner. You love to just simply hang out with me. You are sleeping more peaceably now, more soundly. You are my gauge; if you've stopped worrying as much, so must've I.

You have officially spent 20 years with me today, unofficially even more. You know I wish I could give you millions in gold and billions in diamonds. You also know those things are just things.

You have my heart, sweetie pie. You have my soul, my darling. You are the world's best friend, mother, disinfector, movie-goer, couch-chatter, dog whisperer, crisis manager, comedian and wife.

You are my person of forever.

CHAPTER **54**

# Reports of My Death Are Greatly Exaggerated

My daughter Skye didn't completely think through the message she posted on her friend's Facebook wall last week. They were watching a movie together during a sleepover. At around 2:00 a.m., she was shocked when one of the characters got killed.

HE DIED!!!, she wrote in all caps. Little did she realize, the post showed up in her news feed where family and friends could see it. I commented on it as soon as I realized the possible confusion the next morning. Although I understand the similarities between me and Ryan Phillippe (*http://imdb.to/TV35hB*), I wanted to dispel any fears that perhaps something bad had happened overnight.

Thank you, though, for the flowers from my friends several time zones away in London.

CHAPTER **55**

# My Nutter Brother

MY BLOOD BROTHER Scott gets a pass from me these days for just about any behavior, even destroying Christmas centerpieces.

When he got up and decided to spin Marci's exercise ball on his finger, Taylor tossed her phone into movie mode to record the epic failure. Normally this type of boys-gone-bad behavior would truly annoy me, but deep down, it didn't bother me at all. Maybe it's because he handed over his stem cells a few months ago. Maybe I've become a better person. But probably it's because I knew a good story trumps a dopey snowman made out of fake ice cubes any day.

Speaking of Scott, he handed me what hopefully is the last of the bills from all my brother's and cousin's blood testing. All the incredible fundraising over the summer and fall truly made a difference and covered the medical costs not covered by insurance.

But I think it's important that everyone realizes I did my part too. The $40.00 doctor bill he gave me was for a random scan I didn't know took place. Later that night after giving me the bill, I played poker with all the brothers and cousins that were tested. I won exactly and precisely $40.00. I'm not sure they all appreciated the coincidence, though.

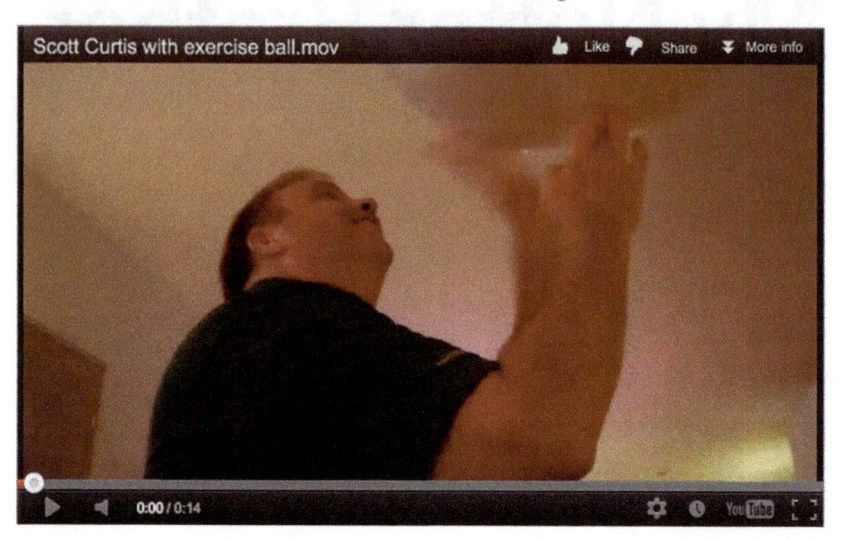

You can watch the devastation here. (http://bit.ly/UXl7Qi)

CHAPTER 56

# Day 100

LET ME CHECK the time. Okay, it's a quarter-to-everything.

At this point on the clock, there's a huge evening-out process which sounds like a night on the town, but is really just the process of making myself even-Steven, even-Rodney. They tried to kill me with chemotherapy, then just at the last second, they resurrected me with my brother's stem cells. Yin and yang.

That was 100 days ago.

I made it through the most critical time, post-transplant. Success or failure seems to be determined by the 100-day milestone. Most of the bad stuff happens during the first 100 days.

It felt like 100 years.

When I look back at last week, I don't think I've progressed so much. When I look back at last month, I know I have. My cool Aunt Roberta says I need to gauge my journey now in months. It feels so much better than clocking myself by days, like I did back in the summer and fall. I just wanted to get out of the hospital, *"Home, where I wanted to roam,"* like *Coldplay* sings.

I contracted diseases in the hospital that I'll spend my life trying to forget. I've caught bugs here at home that little babies get, except with me they linger for weeks. I watch the clock when it's the calendar that begs my attention. I grieve for seemingly silly things that I somehow relate to. I'm sad for Steve Jobs. But I'm also affected by more personal matters like my college trombone buddy Charlie, whose cancer is back. His has the same name as mine used to have, Acute Myeloid Leukemia.

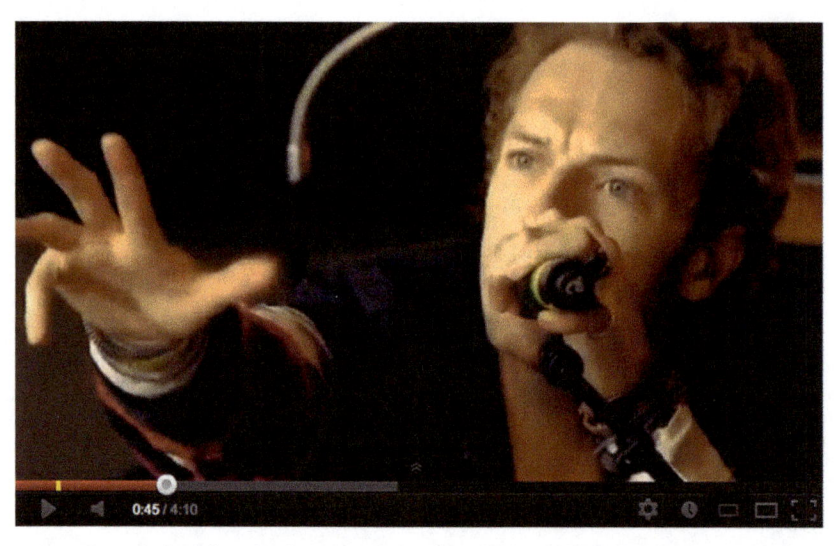

**The Coldplay lads sing Clocks. (http://bit.ly/W0asUj).**

I still give myself shots in the belly and consume 20 pills of different shapes every day. But I'm also exercising now like the "old people," by walking in the mall before it opens. I get irrationally mad at bad drivers these days; life seems too fragile to jeopardize it doing dumb things behind the wheel. Then an angry man flips me off on I-75 and I realize life is too short to get upset at people doing dumb things behind the wheel.

152 • A "Cute" Leukemia

These 100 days have been liberating and weird as all hell. At the same time, I work hard to move past my sickness, then I pop pills that make me remember my predicament. A small bit of a scary rejection disease invades my body and the doctors are pleased. Apparently you want a little bit of it, but no, uh-uh, not too much of it.

The dichotomy in this is gut-changing.

So I take on different themes for myself. One that's worked better than most is "Embrace Life." Oh, it sounds noble and like a philosophy anyone could get behind, but usually its working definition is "Order more pizza" or "Sure, ice cream with whipped topping counts as embracing life, dammit."

The bitter January only has about a week left, then the hallelujah days of February begin melting Michigan, slowly, almost imperceptibly.

My next 100 days will be spent re-creating my own reality, looking and laughing along with the coincidences that raise their heads like our February groundhog friend. I'll also spend them observing myself and wondering what I've become and what I am becoming.

I'm not totally me yet. But I think I have a feel for who he is.

CHAPTER **57**

# Cool or Creepy?

**FACT : T**HIS video—of Scott and me boxing—was shot nine years, a couple houses and several jobs ago.

**FACT :** Just this past fall, I received a bone marrow transplant from my brother Scott.

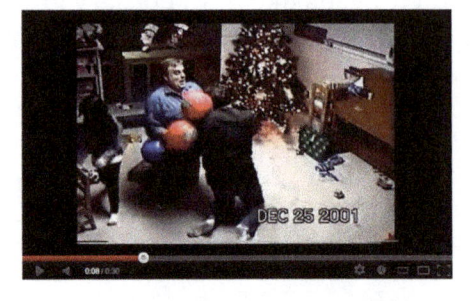

As my daughter Taylor and I were looking at old family movies for a video she was putting together for her sister's birthday, we stumbled across this 30-second clip. Our jaws dropped—really, physically dropped, as we stared at each other in a stunned stupor. Everyone else in our extended family had the same reaction to Marci's seemingly innocuous commentary, while taping us whapping each other. Back then there wasn't even a

See me beat on Scott while Marci channels Nostradamus. (http://bit.ly/W0av2x)

hint of my leukemia or health issues to come in eight-and-a-half years.

I don't believe coincidences are merely random events in our lives. They are occurrences that point to some higher, subtle interconnectedness between all of us. I keep a "Connection Collection" file on my desktop and update it regularly with amazing and simple events that happen to and around me. This is my latest entry in that log.

(For those of you reading this in a paperback book and don't want to bother going online, in the video my wife warns my brother and I "You are each other's transplant, people.")

CHAPTER 58

# The Fighter

It hasn't been easy.

Before I launch into why or what hasn't been easy, I should explain, as an example, that typing the word "easy" took three different attempts. My vision goes in and out at close range. It could be the result of the natural progression of age but I find myself blaming it, among a myriad of other maladies, on the chemicals that—in the past via chemotherapy and now with the 20 pills I take daily—have scrambled my body and to some extent my brain as well.

Yes, I just had to re-read and modify that previous sentence to make sure it contained a shred of sense. Do you see where I am?

It's my new normal, as much as I despise that phrase. I want my old normal back. As I get better, I expect my body to follow a linear progression upwards. Who am I kidding? I demand that progress. I feel like a character in a movie who goes through tremendous turmoil but during the montage scene, two-thirds of the way through, rebuilds and reconstructs his life and comes out the winner.

Sometimes there's a soundtrack to this phase. Generally, though, it's just the weird burbles in my stomach and my wife and kids encouraging me, understanding when all I want to do is sleep. Winter is a good time for the sleep excuse. Rebuilding isn't always being the fighter in the meat locker punching sides of beef.

*(If you don't understand that last sentence you're either very young or don't like movies all that much. Google the sentence if you must, starting with "fighter." The first of 70-some pages will help you. The very last entry at the bottom of page 71 from "ask the meat man dot com" probably won't.)*

I choose or chose the fighting analogy flippantly, but there are parallels. There is a constant war going on in my body called GVHD, which sounds like something in high def. In reality it's called Graft vs. Host Disease and it refers to my brother's blood rejecting my body as its new home. You want a little of that war to happen. And so far, the battlefield has been my skin of all places and my mouth, if you can believe it.

Hey, I'm not writing all this for sympathy. It's just the most honest answer I have to the frequent question "How are you doing?"

This past week of sunshine and almost 60 degree temperatures worked wonders for my mood. My pill-infused tummy even felt a bit better, less chaotic. Then the foot of snow arrived and I was sure it would bury my levity. But so far, no, I am back in training and the montage scene has reached its crescendo.

What the fighter does now, the audience doesn't really know. But nobody buys tickets to comedy-dramas without expecting a few twists along the way towards a warm, satisfying ending.

And by "ending," I mean beginning.

CHAPTER 59

# Tub Thai

M**Y SENSITIVE STOMACH** these days values a few things more than most others. Mellow and mild comfort food is one. A warm bath where my tummy can assume a more weightless state is the other. Not being plagued by gravity's pull can sometimes feel really good in your gut.

I don't know if there's any sound, scientific sense, but my belly generally feels better when I'm in a soothing baby lotion bath.

Given the time I have on my hands and my undeniable predilection toward goofiness, I decided to combine the two. It answers the age-old question: "What do you get when you combine pad thai and a warm soak in the tub?"

This experiment forced me to answer another perplexing question—does the three- second rule apply when you drop one of your chopsticks onto the bath mat? I didn't want to take any chances, so I dipped it into the bath water just to "sanitize" it.

We've all done ridiculous things in our lives. The only difference between you and me is I am willing to share my foibles in writing.

The silly things we do are most memorable and add spice to our lives. They also add noodles to our baths, apparently, if my progress so far is any indication. One of the most rebellious things I did as a youth was go out vandalizing things on Devil's Night.

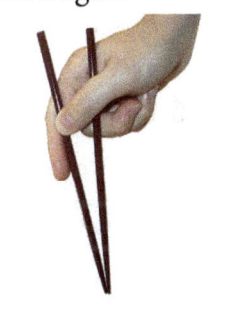

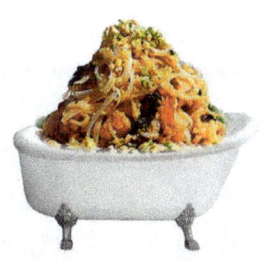

Anyway, my "vandalizing" took the form of rubbing soap on other people's privates ... *oops, spellcheck kicked in ...* other people's private property. I was a sheltered child in some ways, so I was too scared to soap people's windows like the other neighborhood ruffians.

So I rubbed soap all over a homeowner's decorative rock, way out on the outskirts of their lawn. I feel better finally admitting that (unless I already wrote about it, in which case I'm one sad specimen).

My point here is that I am easily entertained. And apparently, it usually centers around cleaning products. Sometimes my health or emotions preclude me from getting excited about much of anything. In this third trimester of winter, you'll have to excuse me if noodles and bubbles send me into a reverie.

CHAPTER **60**

# The International Symbol for Embarrassment

THERE SEEMS TO be some sort of internal threshold that I've crossed. It feels as though I have passed a milestone in my recovery that has allowed me to feel next to normal. Not to pile on the metaphors, but it's as though a switch were flipped and from here on out I'll be gauging wellness by how I feel now, as opposed to when I was sickly.

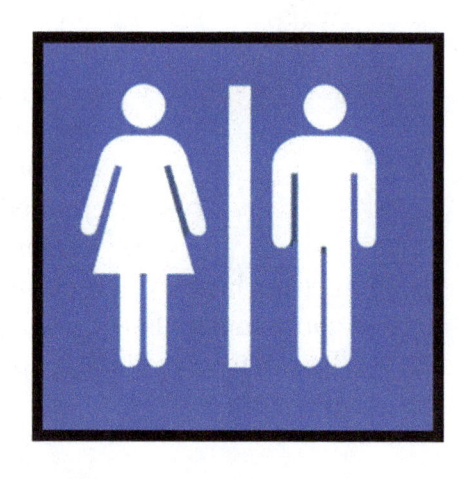

Hopefully.

Hopefully now isn't an aberration. Hopefully our trip to the Pacific Northwest didn't hold a magical elixir of rain and beauty which combined to make me feel better. I don't fancy moving out there for good, although they had amazing coffee drinks.

I almost feel antsy now. I want things to progress rapidly, both in my professional life as well as my health. Specifically, I want to stop taking all these pills, quit giving myself shots in the belly, cease taking nap after nap and, yes, grow a heck of a lot more hair than I've already managed to push out my scalp. All those things will happen in due time. I shouldn't be greedy now that I've accomplished—at least for now—my near-normalcy goal.

And lest you think all is perfect, I'll offer up this one tiny example of how I'm not exactly back to perfection.

My fingernails, mouth and eyes still are giving me fits. The doctors have me on pills for that, too.

When we were in the Portland airport waiting to board the red eye, I took one last quick potty stop. Walking into the abandoned bathroom, I quickly sought out a stall and did my business. If you're a dude reading this, you understand that it's not mandatory that you close your toilet stall if you're just peeing. I heard a guy with dress shoes stomping in. He stopped right behind my stall and then strode back out.

"Hmm, that's odd. Oh, well," were my thoughts, in that order.

I finished up, washed my hands, noted the lack of any urinals and exited the women's room.

Standing outside with her back to me, was the "guy" who'd invaded my session. At least she wouldn't … oh, God, no … yes, I had to sit right behind her on the plane.

I think Marci was wondering why I was speaking so loudly about my vision being blurry as we stowed our luggage and sat down.

In my life, normal and crazy abnormal have fought each other for years. I think I know who's winning.

chapter 60 • 161

## CHAPTER 61

# Following My Heart

MAYBE THERE WAS something in my heart telling me I should return to the hospital. That's probably why this most recent Friday the 13th—a day that began so nicely by meeting one of my favorite baseball stars, Magglio Ordonez—I found myself driving to the emergency room with chest pains.

"There's no way I'm having a heart attack," I kept reassuring myself. But the signs were all there; difficulty breathing, pain in my chest and side, reluctance to admit it was a heart attack, blah, blah, blah.

No, I obviously shouldn't have been driving myself, but my wife and girls were over at the high school and since I was much closer to my destination I thought I shouldn't disturb them. I hopped in the car and took off. Don't try this at home.

I-75 was jammed so I decided on an alternate route. Thankfully it passed right by another emergency room in a sort of Redi-Med building across from Costco. I swung in there.

"Hi," I said to the receptionist. "I am a bone marrow transplant patient with a history of leukemia and blood clots who is experiencing pains in the chest and difficulty breathing." Man, I sounded so professional. "Oh, and I'm on blood thinners, too." I was proud of my ability to succinctly give my history, like a walking/talking medical alert bracelet. But I was also supremely embarrassed.

"This is probably nothing," I assured myself.

They got me checked in immediately and started the testing right away. Thankfully the heart monitor showed no abnormality and the blood tests indicated everything was okay. That didn't help the look on my daughters' faces, though, when I saw them later on. Seeing their fear, after I had been reassuring them over and over again throughout the past year, made me realize yet again how my battle wasn't just being waged for myself.

What new fresh hell were they experiencing?

From the walk-in ER, I took an ambulance ride downtown in the bumpiest vehicle I've been in since, I don't know, the old Ford pickup truck on the farm in North Dakota I used to visit when I was a kid. Down at the "real hospital," they kept prodding and poking and taking blood until a 1:00 a.m. ultrasound proved it was only pericarditis, a swelling of the sac surrounding the heart. More than likely it was brought on by my artificially low immune system or my previous bout with leukemia. The treatment? Motrin.

Seriously.

That previous sentence was longer than the amount of sleep I got that night, but I was happy to go home the next day, relieved that, at least for me, the stress was over. But I think in my family's eyes, this opened old wounds that had only recently begun to scar over.

We've spoken about it individually and, bless all their hearts, they don't want me worrying about them. My biggest concern is obviously with their personal states of mind.

We run the risk in the Curtis family of worrying too much about each other and not enough about ourselves, so somehow I need to shatter this. I know when I'm a year, two years,

chapter 61 • 163

five and ten years removed from all this, it will be easier for them to not live on pins and hypodermic needles. But I want that for them now, right freakin' now.

And I'm sure what they want most, right freakin' now, is for me to stop worrying about them.

CHAPTER **62**

# Mr. Compassion

MY FAMILY IS sick. Today is my lucky day.

Yes, I realize those first few sentences go together like pizza and warm tap water, but for a guy who's been taken care of all these months, it's my turn to give back.

A sniffly wife? "There there, honey, what can I fetch you?"

A tired, groaning daughter? "Hey, girl, would you like some yummy Jell-O?"

It's not like the sum total of all their pills would even come close to matching my current daily dosage. Heck, I take pills to counteract the other pills I take to help me consume the first ones.

I'm happy being the helper. Oh sure, they're sick, I get that. But right now it makes me feel better. I think I need a shrink.

It could be just a matter of moments before I come down with what they have. My immune system is still being kept low with all the pills from a few paragraphs ago. But in this sweet spot where I reside right now, I get to play the compassionate caregiver. Pay no attention to that sneeze I just stifled.

My ladies mean everything to me. If you read my first book you'll remember they're even more special than frozen coffee. Turning the tables and looking on them with sympathy and benevolence is a gas. They can see the caring and nurturing in my eyes, much like they've had in their own eyes since about forever ago.

I'm a good person again. My joy in their illness proves it.

CHAPTER **63**

# Heavy Sigh

**I HAD TO** bag out of helping my daughter with her Relay for Life team.

I had to miss my other daughter's 24-hour music marathon.

I wasn't there for my best buddy Bob's brother's funeral.

And when a good friend drove a couple hundred miles with his daughters to surprise me, I wasn't there either.

I'm back in the hospital. Yes, it's for yet another side effect on the growing list of zany things that happen to Rodney due to his recovery. I am feeling a lot better now, but what makes me sickest is that I didn't tell anybody except my closest family, simply due to misplaced pride.

I'll start from the beginning.

I was pretty lethargic for the two weeks following that incident with the swollen heart lining, pericarditis. When I had one too many low grade fevers, Marci packed me up one night and drove me down to Karmanos. We didn't even wake up our daughters since I didn't want to scare them (something they might never forgive me for). Test after test, poke after poke showed nothing out of the ordinary until someone got it in their head to do a CAT scan of my chest.

BINGO.

Remember that lining around my heart? You and I are supposed to have less than an ounce of fluid between it and the heart. After the scan showed far more than that, the doctors stuck a long tube and needle into my chest and started draining the excess. And draining, and draining, and draining ...

When all of it finally dripped out—over the course of three days—it measured about a liter and a half. I took a lousy photo with my camera phone. That's not even all the liquid that came out. There was even more heart juice in other vials. The heart wall isn't designed to hold so much. Generally speaking, a couple tablespoons of liquid is enough for the ol' ticker.

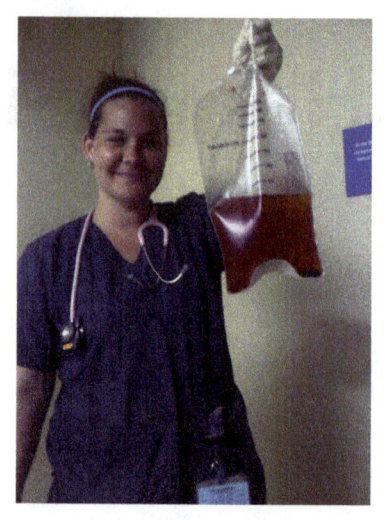

**Nurse Erin was left holding the bag.**

If it filled up suddenly, I would have definitely felt it. Apparently it slowly grew over the course of a few weeks. All of these medical issues lately are caused by Graft vs. Host Disease. Apparently that's a good thing; I'm told this shows my new system has pluck and won't shy away from a good fight. The doctors like to see that. Although having two sons fighting it out, Mom's probably gonna turn the car around and not take us to the zoo.

That's what happened, but it doesn't explain or excuse me from not talking about it. I think part of my problem is disease overload. I don't want to keep talking, over and over again about the things I've been having to deal with. But there's more. I want to feel normal and human and not look at myself as a work in progress any more. I'm tired of being a poster boy.

A story from my distant past kind of illustrates my point. I was walking our dog down the block when she yanked at the leash and pulled me to the cement, scraping my knee. I was crying and just as I pulled myself up, a carload of my neighbors drove right by me. I threw on a shit-eating-grin and waved like a ninny at them. I'm sure, in retrospect, they probably saw my dog pull me down and could maybe even see my tears and snotty nose. But I didn't want to look like anything bad had happened to me, to feel vulnerable or out of control. I wanted to look normal. I didn't want to be the center of attention for something bad. I was embarrassed.

Sounds all too familiar.

So I didn't tell people about this latest heart-rending travesty. It's weird because I really try to always be open and honest with everybody. And that's the thing; by being so above-board with everything else, I have gotten so much support and encouragement.

I shied away this time. Sometimes I'm just a barrel of contradictions.

CHAPTER **64**

# A Year and Today

A **YEAR AGO** this morning, I woke up early, drove to Michigan State University and gave a guest lecture.

A year ago today, I golfed in the late morning with my buddy.

A year ago today, we ate late-lunch pizza and joked about nearly everything.

A year ago today, in the early evening hours, my family's world got sucked into an insane parallel universe where 40 percent of my body was infested with leukemia and the future, suddenly, had no up or down.

We dealt. We relied on the kindness of strangers. We somehow found *down* first, then *up*. So many incredible people showed up and did the most incredible and simple things. As I drank chemo for breakfast, followed by a healthy bone marrow lunch, we saw the black hole shrink and the white whole expand.

I invited the mystical and spiritual in for a party. God and Buddha danced with Mohammed and Jesus. Mother Mary smiled off in the corner, and even Shiva showed up. White light, army flame-throwers and cute, tiny blue bubbles went to work.

Daughters dove and acted, performed and scored. Family ate surprise dinners left on our porch. Sometimes we faked it and maked it. We even dared to travel. Sure, a setback here and there, but the only thing we didn't mourn the lack of was leukemia. Gone. Probably for good. Or evil.

Today—as I was fixing my daughters' breakfasts and packing their lunches—Taylor said, "Hey, happy one year." It's not written on a calendar, nor had we discussed the date, but it was stamped somewhere on her mental album of last year.

Today, I received a phone call. A bone marrow symposium this fall in Atlanta loves my t-shirt design and asked if I would mind being flown down to photograph their event.

There's pizza in my future today.

Happy today.

CHAPTER 65

# Oh, Steroids

W HEN YOU CAN'T sleep and it's 4:00 in the morning, there's usually a reason, like your mind is racing or you're in some type of pain—mental or physical—or there's something unexplainable bothering you. Of course, it could be the steroids.

These lovely, magical, insane chemicals are tailor-made to keep the bad diseases at bay and fix me up right good so I can hop back into the ring. But they also help me do other things like eat insane amounts of food, experience temporary diabetes, poop like a porpoise and now sit awake at night trying to think of funny-sounding aquatic animals that I share similar digestive predilections with.

(Just for the record, I scratched "crap like a crab," "s#@t like a seahorse" and "have an enema like an anemone." You're welcome.)

I tend to think weird thoughts when everybody else is asleep. Like, if I sign up on the Timex, Longines or Swatch forums, do I automatically go on a watch list?

*(Again, you're welcome.)*

Then I hit a wall and can't decide whether I'm writing in third person, first person or alien. I stare at the screen wondering who wrote those previous paragraphs and remember there's a bed upstairs waiting for me. I make a note to myself to never write something this banal and make another note to myself to look up the word banal.

A bird chirps and it pisses me off because I detect a certain sarcasm in his one-character tweet.

Minutes pass between words as vzabsuuudjkldjkh zcxm …

CHAPTER **66**

# The Traumas of June

IN THE DREAM, I was panicking. I had uprooted the whole family to move back to Midland so I could work at a small startup news organization with an uncertain future. Do you know those times, within dreams, where you start to realize you have no background information? It's like you've parachuted into a plot of a long-running story and you're supposed to pick up right where the action is.

We were in a rickety building, crowded with people from my past. I was supposed to be the informal head of the household but really, it was my wife. It was late at night; my job was starting the next day and I had no idea what I was doing. Very familiar dream theme there, Rodney; -20 points for lack of creativity.

As I'm freaking out in the dream, I reach out for Marci's help and she's there, comforting me. As I wake up, there she is again, very much concerned and probably ready to call 911. I was moaning and thrashing around in bed, in real life. And when she asks what's happening I say I'm sorry, but I can't explain. Then reality hits and I say, "Oh, wait, that was really dumb."

Instead of having a coronary, I was having a corollary.

Two Junes ago, my family was in upheaval as my 25-year career in journalism was being swiped out from underneath me. Last June, we all know what happened as, again with circumstances beyond my control, an insidious disease caused my family pain and suffering. My week-long hospitalization this June, well, you get the picture.

I think there's some sort of post-traumatic stress factor working its way through my system now. Even as my sweet wife and I sit up smiling in the dark about the sillier aspects of the dream, I begin to see the connections between a ridiculous manufactured nocturnal storyline and the very real upheaval that we've gone through.

One was drama, the other, trauma.

And here is where the connections are leading me. Here is where we've arrived. I'm glad my girls' school is so close to done for the year. My family needs—no, requires—a break from the hard-charging push. But I think it's even simpler. I think it's what Marci was saying to me as she was waking me from the dream that somehow combined all our Junes into one, the co-seismic turmoil of journalism and cancer.

Just breathe. Take a deep breath. Relax. There is no elephant in the living room that we're all avoiding. It's just my family's need to de-stress.

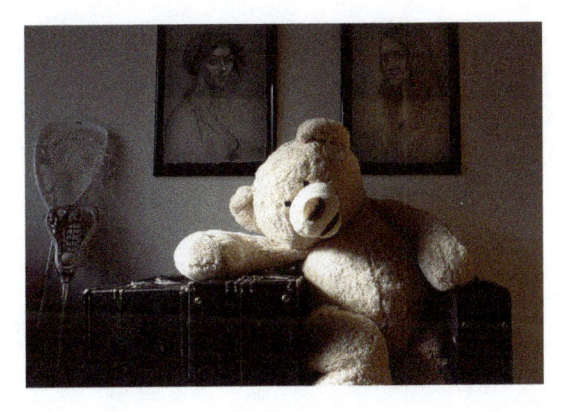

Although, when I woke again this morning, instead of an elephant, there was a giant bear with a bunch of baritones in the homework room. And if you all can see this too, it means I'm reasonably awake and not in a bizarre dream world anymore.

It just means Skye is handing out instruments before band camp. At least that explains the baritones. The bear is still a wild uncertainty.

Exhale.

CHAPTER **67**

# Interlacing Threads

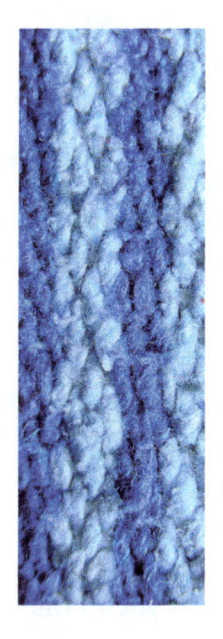

I **FIND MYSELF** ever-increasingly blown away by the power of the weird tapestry that's woven us all into its warp. I didn't make it to my high school reunion last weekend. Nor did I attend my college reunion last fall. Both would have been fascinating, but I was preoccupied with my health. I know, where are my priorities?

But one of the side effects of reunions and frightening diseases is people tend to reconnect with you. That and chicken dinners. There have been some long-ago friends that have resurfaced, at least for a while. And I've gotten closer still with friends that have been there all along. When a best buddy's brother died, I got a huge hug and was told simply, "I'm glad you're still around."

"Me too," I said.

A couple guys I went to kindergarten with checked in. One I had known since the 70s, the other loaned me money after college so I could hitchhike around Ireland. We've talked on and off since, with perhaps years in between that separated our conversations. I don't exactly know how all of it happens, but there's always a new or old friend knocking on my electronic door. Often it's exactly when I need to hear something important or say something profound … or so I think.

My incredibly non-jealous wife smiles when former crushes, mine or theirs, say hi. Yes, they've all been female. But I had been estranged, for lack of a more creative word, from a guy who seemed both twisted and braided to me, like my alter ego. We got back together when things were dire last summer. He's visited and sent me insane messages that made me laugh like we were kids again. He even tried to get me down to the Caribbean on an all-expenses-paid trip. Who says cancer is all bad?

I've been lucky, due to the latest reunion round, to chat with some of the people I hung out with in high school. They were the types who were more on the side—in classes, maybe a party or two. It's been amazing. Whether it's the wine impresario, now in St. Louis, who I missed many opportunities with in high school, or the always good and kind band mate who still lives back in the 'hood, I have benefitted from our threads overlapping once again in life's rich tapestry.

Last night and today, via the Internet's weave, I bumped into a casual friend from the horizon who'd been hurting for years. A lost partner and enough bad news to last a lifetime gave her the ability to reach out and offer me the opportunity to give back a thread to the loom that ever plaits.

"Hopefully," I said to her, "you can find other experiences and people who pull you towards them magnetically, until the realization that we're all interconnected smacks you in the face."

I get. I give. Back and forth we all interlace.

CHAPTER **68**

# Back in the Saddle (Again?)

"Don't worry, Jeffrey," I told my buddy while we devoured smokehouse grub at the trendy Royal Oak meat market. "There's no way I'm going to call you, moaning 'shoot my wedding for me.'"

Jeffrey Sauger (*http://bit.ly/TV33pS*) had shot two previous gigs for me when I was taken out of life's rodeo because of the now-familiar cancer thing. He and Rob Widdis (*http://bit.ly/TV33pU*) have come through on either a few weeks' or a few days' notice, depending on how quickly I was tossed from the bucking bronco.

I got bucked, all right.

But this time I was staying on my ride. This time I was not going to plant my face in the dirt and watch, ringside from the hospital bed, as another fun wedding slipped past me.

But then all that smokehouse meat I ate caught up to me. Or the organic vegetables. Or the peach that maybe wasn't quite ripe. Or maybe it was just another one of those blah, blah, blahs that love to buck with me during recovery.

When I woke up Saturday morning feeling oogy, I was thinking I'd have to go back on my word and call Jeffrey/Rob to see if they could spring into action, this time with just a few hours' notice.

But I gutted it out. There was actually an internal struggle (in more ways than one) pitting me vs. me.

Happily, I won.

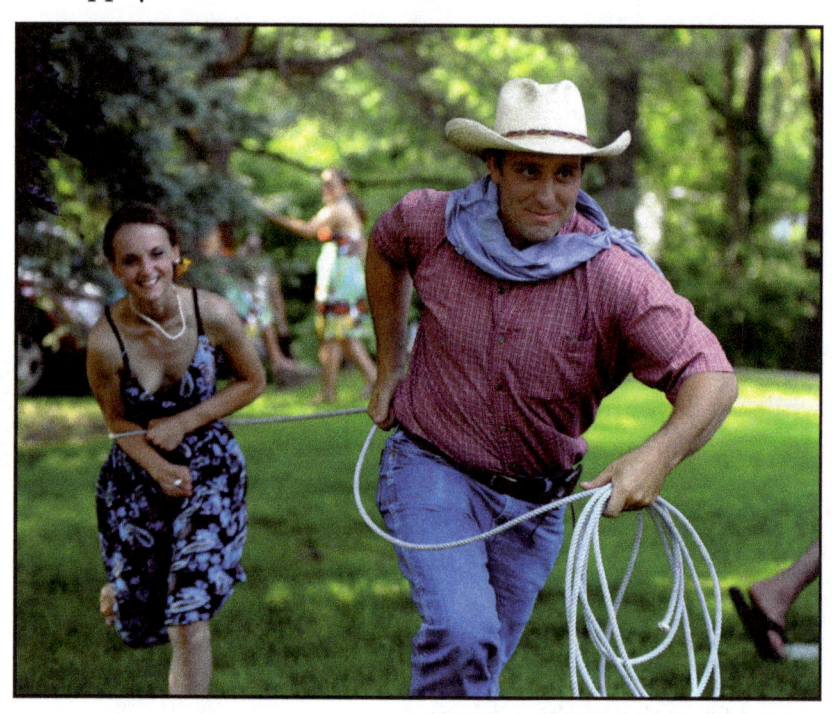

Our family friends, the Greens, were having a hoedown reception in their backyard—contrasting the formal wedding—of their son to their new daughter-in-law. The young couple love animals and I happily was lassoed in to shoot the roundup.

There were miniature cows, tiny goats, ducks, chickens, dogs, a pig (but it was called "dinner") and lots of humans. This is a normal occurrence at the Green's home. You have to believe me when I say none of the animals were only there for that special day, except for the pig (and some of the humans). Their house and land is the coolest in all of Troy; they didn't even use their barn because it was far too hot on the high 90-degree Saturday. Suburban cowboys.

The day was made even more special by the addition of my ranch-hand daughter, Taylor. At 15, she was the last remaining member of the family who hadn't earned some coin helping out at weddings. Since Abby Green is "her besty," she was glad to be my photo assistant. The first thing we heard when we walked into the bridal room, where everyone was busy getting ready, was a loud "TAYLOR!"

She thought she was in trouble, but no, one of the Green kids needed her hair re-done. I checked back in later to find Taylor doing another sister's toenails. "Tay, honey, I need you to take pictures, too," I said.

In lieu of an answer, she flicked the camera's preview button to show me what she'd shot already. "That's pretty darn good, girl!"

She went back to painting nails.

Seriously, she had several shots already that I wished I'd taken. She went on to have a whole herd of really nice photos. And having her there to cover for me, when the heat got to be too much, was critical.

Don't worry Jeffrey and Rob, if you're reading this, you won't get stampeded by a teen girl.

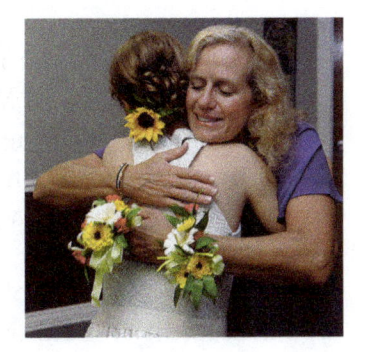

Yet.

No, all kidding aside, it's tremendous to know there are great people all around me who have my back before, during and after weddings. But mostly in life.

This ain't my first rodeo. Thankfully, it ain't my last.

chapter 68 • 181

CHAPTER **69**

# Dumb & More Dummer

THERE HAVE BEEN times in my life I've been stupid. I mean, grand-scale, thinking-outside-the-box dumb. Hard to believe, I know.

No, I'm not referring to when I couldn't get my car started, early one morning up in Midland, so I jumped it with the van, pulled out, closed the garage door and went to work. The scared-out-of-her-wits phone call from my wife a few hours later asking why the van was running in a closed garage still terrifies me.

That was a mistake. Epic, yes, but it wasn't planned. The type of stupidity I'm thinking about involves me making a conscious decision to do dumb.

But boy, both times I did were insanely fun. Yes, I've only been purposefully preposterous twice in my life. If anyone knows of other times, shhhhh!

Number one on my list is "skeetching." You probably haven't heard much about skeetching since, oh I don't know, the 1970s. If you are under 18, you might want to go surf for something less inappropriate like catsthatlooklikehitler.com or cracked.com.hair today Okay grownups, to skeetch you need two things: a car and a very snowy road. Uh, you need three things: stupidity, a car and a very snowy road.

The driver of the car, knowingly or unwittingly, drives down said snowy road while the skeetcher grabs onto the bumper and slip-slides away. Kids back in the ridiculous years of the 70s would sometimes even pretend to help a stranded motorist by pushing them out of a snowy patch, then hold tight as the car drove away.

The definition of dumb.

In my case, a group of my friends decided that one very dark and snowy winter's night was the ideal time to jeopardize our futures. The Pleasant Ridge cops were known for their systematic cruising and once they came by your street, they assuredly wouldn't be back again for hours. We watched and waited for them to make their pass but that night they never did.

One of us got to be the "responsible" designated driver, while the others held onto the rear of the car and crouched, bent over, or even laid down for the duration. Inches of snow separated us from death or road rash. It was hysterical.

Then we got the bright idea to "Indiana Jones it" and try to push all the others off. I remember holding on with one hand, skidding along the street, all the while pushing/pulling and punching my buddies to get them to fall off first. Sometimes we'd even wrap our bodies around each other and let go, thus pulling both parties off to a declared draw.

Morons.

God, but it was fun.

It took another 10 years before I signed on to something almost as insane. And this time I brought my wife along for the ride.

In New Hampshire, some friends of friends of friends were thinking about opening a riding stable that catered to more adventurous horse enthusiasts. Would we, they wanted to know, help them experiment? And oh, by the way, it would be at night.

Let's see, enormous animals, a moonless New Hampshire evening and galloping? Sure, sign us up.

The thought was that horses know the trails they ride day in and month out. Why not take riders along these same trails at nighttime?

Why not?

There's not a lot to report. Really. If you've ever ridden on Space Mountain you may remember zipping through mostly darkness, whipping this way and that, not knowing when things would end. Imagine doing that, except not on a track, or with seat belts, or a mega insurance policy backed by years of precision testing.

Yeah, imagine that. We were trotting along the blind backwoods when suddenly the horses came to the place where they normally run. Giddy-up. They took off like shooting stars, streaking through the night—although with far, far less illumination.

And that was our nighttime horseback ride. Later, the moon rose and it was actually quite beautiful. Our guides circled back to make sure, mostly, that we were all there. And later, we drove home shaken to the very core of our beings with wobbly thighs and saddle sores. Wow, that was awesome.

Those were the two most idiotic things I've ever done.

Until now.

Way, way back when I didn't have to check in with my doctors every week or two, I packed my summer with travel. I was sure everything would go smoothly so I figured why not travel to the wilds of Canada, then down to slightly less wild North Carolina. I ignored the distance from me, at any given point, to a bone marrow specialist, or a hospital, or even a doctor.

I may as well have migrated to Marrakesh for the reaction I got from my doctors. "What if something goes wrong?" they wanted to know.

"Uh, maple syrup's good on cuts, eh?"

I think I must've batted my eyelashes and made my best puppy dog face because they agreed to my travel, as long as I stopped in for a full exam before, between and after the trips.

I'll admit, laying in my bed at the very tip of the Bruce Peninsula jutting into Lake Huron, I realized I was hours away from any help if the unforeseeable were to bump in the night. It made me kind of nervous. Not nervous as in dragging from a car or screaming, equine-style, through the night. But I inhaled and exhaled more calmly as the vacation came to an end. Although, Canadian health care is awfully darn good and affordable!

I'm heading to North Carolina next and am hoping for snowless roads and horseless paths. No, traveling isn't stupid, per say. But wandering far from care when my sole job these days is to heal, well, maybe it's not the brightest decision.

Never mind the quicksand, Mr. Livingstone; isn't the jungle lovely?

I'm bound to do more dumb things in my life. Determined, actually. And surely more idiotic things I've done will pop up in my memory, or through reminders from those unfortunate enough to have endured them with me.

And kids, if you're still reading, don't try any of this at home.

CHAPTER 70

# California Dreaming

I**N CERTAIN TIMES** in my life, dreams play smaller or bigger roles in my everyday. I think they pop up, sometimes, when I'm not necessarily looking for their guidance. But when dreamy things start clustering together, I need to open my head and listen.

This latest jag of dream sensitivity began when we were outside of New York City. Staying the night in a high-rise hotel, we were awakened by a 2:30 a.m. fire alarm. Some yahoo had hung their wet clothes from their room's sprinkler head and when the weight broke it off, water poured out everywhere. An hour and a half later we were all allowed back in and my daughters were greeted with a message from their friend back in Troy.

"Be careful. I dreamed the hotel you're staying in had an emergency," he said. Apparently this isn't an unusual occurrence with this guy. I can't wait to sit down and hear more about his precognitions.

Earlier this week I was reading an article in one of my favorite magazines, The Sun (*http://bit.ly/TV35xQ*). It was an interview and they were talking about paying attention to your nighttime stories, but not necessarily taking them literally. Obviously, soon afterward, I had a very vivid dream, part of it devoted to Marci being angry with me.

I tried to make sense of it on a gut level or figuratively, but nothing really bubbled up making any sense, (and how could it, really? Who could be mad with little ol' me?). The next day, as my mom, Taylor, our cousin and I jumped out of the van at the airport, Marci asked if we had our passports. Since we were just taking off to California, we didn't need them. But she got angry and was sure I'd told her at home I had them. I was just going to use my license and Taylor, her school ID.

Had no dream forewarned me of her anger, I would've maybe lashed back. We don't fight a lot, she and I, thankfully. This outburst on her part could very well be my fault, too, for misunderstanding her earlier at home. I like to blame my forgetfulness on the ever-decreasing amount of steroids I'm taking. As my old high school chemistry teacher used to say when one of us didn't turn in our homework, "Any excuse is good in a storm."

On the plane out here, Taylor and our cousin Meredith popped another piece into my latest jigsaw dream awareness. Several years back, both of them had the exact same dream. They were up in heaven and each was searching for a multi-colored backpack. There was nothing

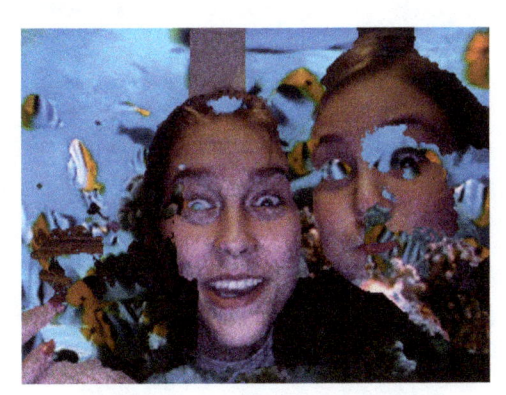

**Taylor and Meredith created this funky dreamscape portrait a while back.**

chapter 70   •   187

around them, in each of their dreams, but when they found the pack, they put in on their backs and carried it with them.

Jung or Freud or any modern day hack could probably interpret that dream forever and a day. But both of them having such a specific dream, separately, was more intriguing to me.

The way we're synchronized with each other or how some things happen simultaneously has always blown my mind. The incredibly mysterious stuff that happens all around us, like dreams coming true, brings such richness and joy to my life. I think it's partly because I like knowing that there's so much more out there, maybe even right under our noses.

That comforts me. I like that the universe or God or the natural world is messing with me. I love knowing that we don't know. A dream glimpse behind the curtain doesn't reveal Oz trying to pull the wool over our eyes, but instead a profound and exciting bag of infinite possibilities.

It's still early in the day, but I can't wait to tumble toward sleep again tonight.

CHAPTER **71**

# Worldwind

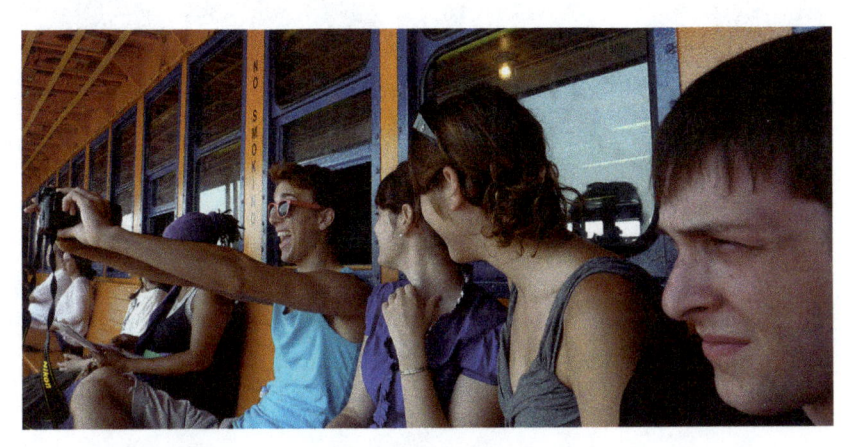

**Tony, Skye, Taylor and Jon have fun on the Staten Island Ferry. Well, at least the first three had some fun.**

A TALE OF two summers tells my story. Last summer, I was kept closed up in hospitals, fighting for my very life, albeit with a smile on my face (mostly). This summer, I decided it was best if I threw myself out into the world in a whirlwind. A *world*wind is more apropos.

Canada, North Carolina, New York City and Los Angeles. Stops in the middle for Philly and D.C. Sure, why not?

There's a rational part of me that says I need to take things a little slower. "Wasn't I just in the hospital as recently as June?" it asks, knowing the answer.

"Yes," I reply, "but that makes it even more imperative that I capture the fish ... You know, 'carpe carp.'"

"Ugh," we both reply.

Honestly, I didn't want another summer to race by while I sat on the sidelines. Sure, I could've taken things a bit slower and in truth, I did for most of June and will again now that August has entered the picture.

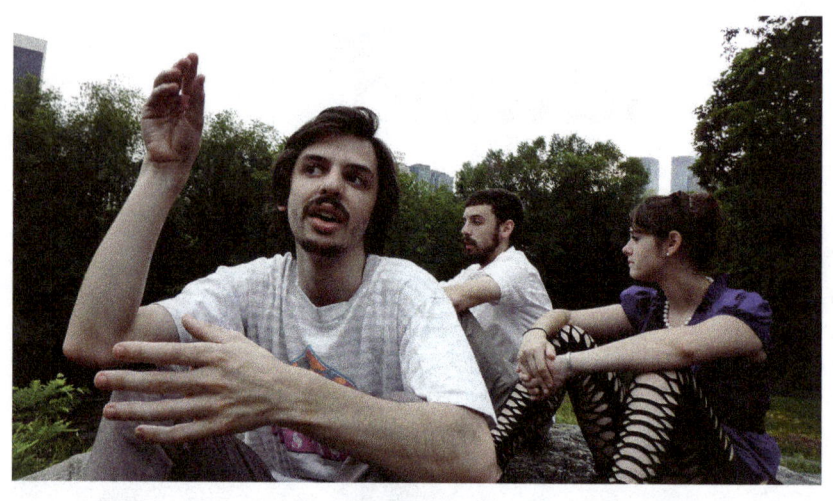

*Hanging out in Central Park with cousins Ben and Tim (and Skye with her post-punk leggings).*

We traveled in different groups this past month, our family splitting up and reassembling. Ohio and Chicago also made appearances, but not on my itinerary. Some people over the years have wondered why the members of my family sometimes take different trips. We wonder why some people *don't* take different trips.

Two of our traveling companions had never experienced the charge of New York. One's a firefighter and Beatles fan, the other, an actor and fashionista. What a perfect Mecca for both. Imagine! Another of our wayfarers had never been to California. We had no choice but to remedy that and since my brother and sister-in-law live there, our rent was insanely cheap.

This is a good place to insert something that's been on my mind for over a year. Many, many folks contributed financial help to our family last summer when things were scary. Even though I probably don't need to say this, all of our traveling has been done on the cheap, like we've done since forever. We hunt for great airfare, find tremendous hotel deals (or stay with family and friends) and avoid restaurants that don't post their menus out front.

I share this because I don't want anyone to think we're squandering their resources. I've been told over and over again I shouldn't feel sorry or guilty for this. I'm sorry; I feel guilty.

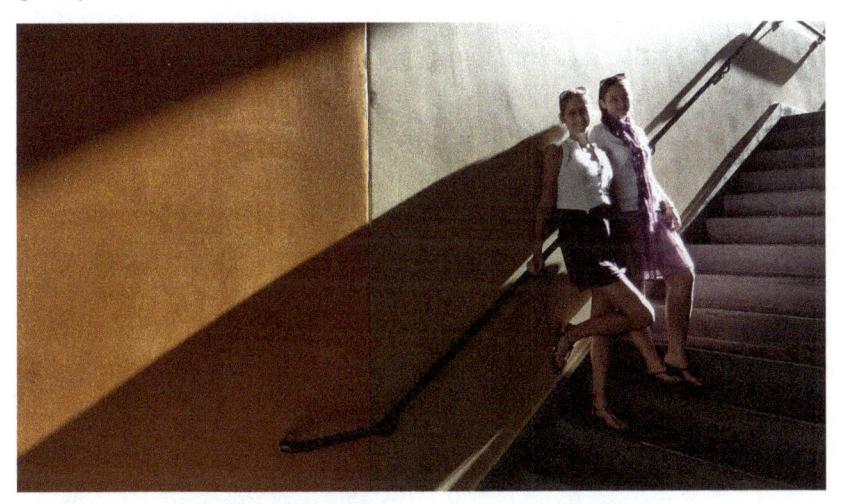

**Taylor and Meredith pause for a Kodak moment at the Kodak Theatre in Hollywood.**

Enough about that. Some wonderful snippets pop up in my head as I scroll through the memories of last month. The greatest one happened on the subway in NYC. My Lady Macraes are very friendly, even with strangers. In supposedly one of the most unfriendly places in an allegedly unfriendly city, sitting across from me was each of my family members chatting with a random stranger. Taylor had engaged a woman from Greece in a discussion about her kids. Marci was talking to a woman from Brooklyn about the heat. Skye was talking to someone about fashion.

It was so fascinating to me, that I remarked to our buddy Jon that everyone in our family had made a friend. At that point, a random woman sitting next to us chimed in, "I

chapter 71 • 191

noticed that. You know, my family is very sociable but I'm just not. They always meet people everywhere but I'm shy. I'm Denise, what's your name?"

There must have been something in the air, humidity maybe. It broke down all of the cold, gruff New Yorker stereotypes and for a brief moment, until our next stop, we were all connected.

In California I played the good little transplant patient and stayed out of the sun for the most part. Oh sure, there were times when I slathered on SPF 50 sunscreen and slipped into my big brother's pool for a few minutes. But when the gang went out someplace sunny, I stayed behind. I saw four movies during my week there and didn't feel like I missed a thing.

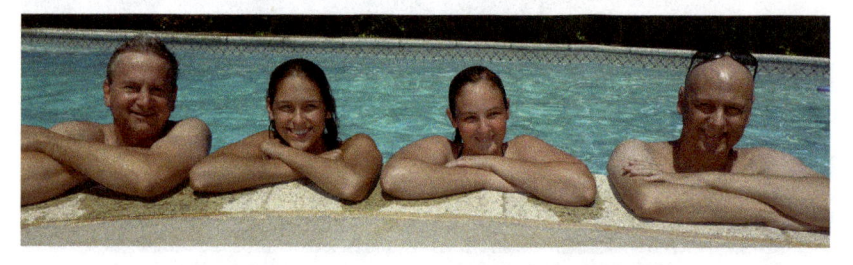

**Damn the torpedoes; if this is Cali, I'm going pool-hopping (but only for a few minutes with enough sunscreen to cover a submarine). Dean, Taylor and Meredith joined me and my SPF 50 oil slick."**

And that's huge. In certain respects, I feel like I'm missing out on life. Not having a job and having to report to a doctor every few weeks leads me to feel like I'm out of step with the rest of society. Then my brain kicks in with the rationalizations, telling me this allows me much more time with my daughters and wife. Valuable time spent with the women I love is incalculable. Then and there, the biggie of all justifications kicks in.

This is all happening for a reason.

Do I believe it? Sometimes, yes I do.

CHAPTER **72**

# These Are My People

IMAGINE BEING IN a room where everyone has had the same shared experience. Some had it decades ago, a few had it less than a year ago, like you. Now imagine a whole conference—a symposium, if you will—where room after room of people speak your language, know what you've gone through and show you, simply by being there, that normal life continues on.

That's exactly what the past four days presented me with. Celebrating a Second Chance at Life, sponsored by bmtinfonet.org (*http://bit.ly/VN2Yno*) threw so much positive energy my way, I didn't even notice I was sleep-deprived and running on Atlanta's fuel, Coca-Cola. Meeting person after person who dealt with cancer and a bone marrow transplant was one of the best experiences I've had over the past year.

Whether it was the organizers of the event, some of whom were marrow recipients, or attendees like the young guy wearing a skull and crossbones bandana, or even the nutty evangelical who tried everything to make his doctors laugh, all of us dealt with the same exact thing. When you've been dangled over the abyss, it's great to know others have hung out there too.

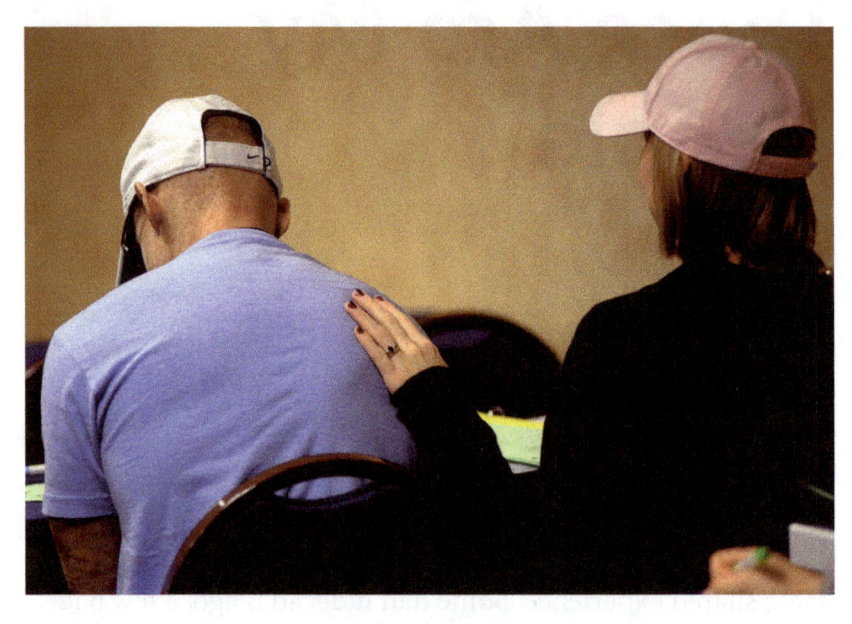

The scenes of intimacy, like the wife constantly scratching her husband's GVHD ravaged back, reminded us that the true heroes in all of this weren't us. They were the caregivers who sat bedside or took on single-parenting duties or cried alone, late at night. There was even a ceremony honoring our caregivers. I picked up a **HERO** bracelet for my wife.

Throughout the seminar, I was known both as the official photographer and a survivor. At the end, there were many tears during my slideshow and no, it wasn't because I had done such a lousy job. Those accolades were wonderful, but the real benefit to me was my ability to pop into one conference room after another. While I was snapping photos and making sure to show every single presenter, I got caught up in their discussions and PowerPoints. I came away with tons of information about myself, including why, Dear God, were my eyes all watery when I was supposedly suffering from dry eye?

There were statistics, facts and studies showing amazing longevity, including how one day soon my chances of getting cancer will be pretty much like everyone else's. There was even some secretive, back-alley talk about new, incredible clinical trials that eliminated certain cancers altogether with just one pill or injection.

Early on, within the first few hours, I told someone "These are my people." I heard the phrase echoed another time during the day then at night, when a fellow leukemia survivor and transplantee was one of the featured singers. She told the crowd the same thing. "These are my people."

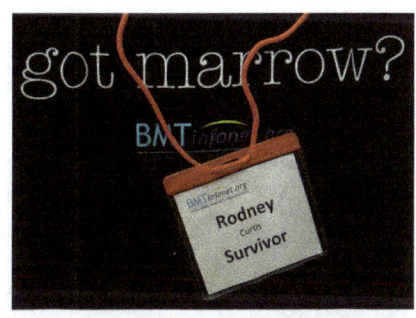

**The organizers even allowed me to design the t-shirt.**

I've belonged to a lot of groups, associations and loose-knit organizations over the years. After the past weekend, I am honored and privileged to be a part of this merry band. Yes, the membership dues were steep and the initiation rituals sucked, but I am guaranteed lifetime access to the fitness center. And that's going to be a mighty long time.

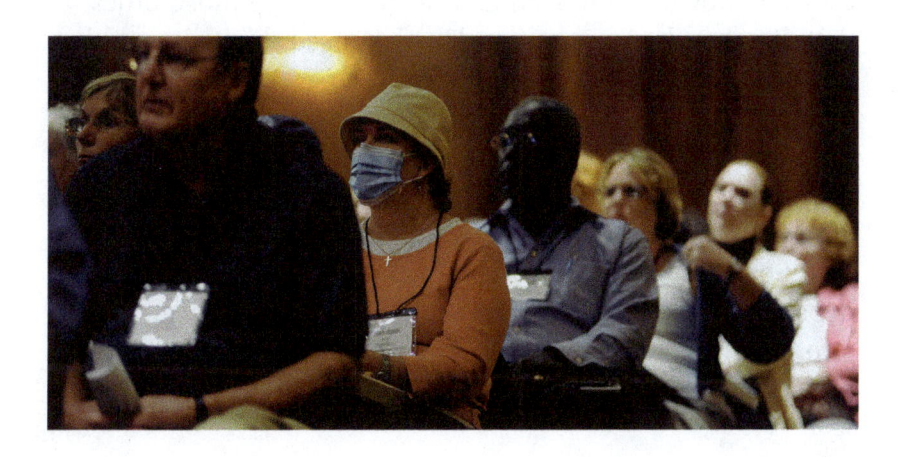

chapter 72 • 195

CHAPTER **73**

# This One's on the House

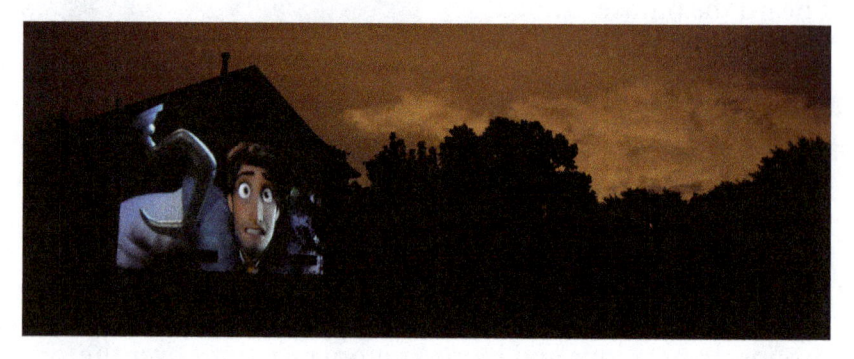

**I WASN'T IN** the mood, a few weeks ago, to show a movie on the side of our house. I've done so a few times in the past, born from a crazy notion that bored into my brain while mowing our lawn. The last time we did the "drive-in" movie was moments before I found out about my cancer. We were also shut down by the authorities—the buzzing mosquitoes that dive-bombed our ears and any exposed skin they could find.

But my daughters kept pushing me to "do the house-movie thing," so I agreed and told them to invite their friends. One thing I've cemented in my mind over this long and slow recovery is to do stuff that makes my family happy. I'm not talking about being a friend instead of a father, although I think that debate has the wrong parameters. I need to facilitate and be a strong advocate for my daughter's growth. That sounds much better than being a pushover.

There are books and blogs about how a father should behave. I'm certain if I looked, there'd be advice on every side of every issue, whether the dad was coming off a layoff, a disease or both. But I have to go with my gut. Even if sometimes my gut is radically wrong and forcibly clouding my judgment, while it digests the steroids and nine other daily drugs I'm on.

I make mistakes all the time, like when our daughter's friends were over and wanted to be treated like family, so I made them help clean the house. It's funny in retrospect, but I was a jerk about it at the time.

I also get it right sometimes, like showing Tangled (<u>http://imdb.to/TV35xY</u>) on a vinyl-sided screen with popcorn and lots of friends.

They know I'm trying. I know they're trying. Sometimes all the trying is trying.

It'll only be a few more ticks of the teen clock until the daughters have moved on to college, careers and kids of their own. I need to remind myself to turn away from the computer and listen to the conversation. And most importantly, when a crazy, unusual request is tossed my way, I need to do my best and catch it.

That's free advice. Just like the movie, it's on the house.

CHAPTER **74**

# Here's to a Year

Yet another year has gone by and I still haven't learned the difference between buffalo and bison, bisque and chowder, the EU and the EC, or Rimsky-Korsakov and a Sikorsky or Kalashnikov.

But I can certainly tell the difference between the me now and the me who left the hospital 365 days ago as a new man, literally. My marrow wasn't my own nor was my blood type the same. I used to be A positive, now I'm O positive. Or vice versa, I'm not positive. I'll text my brother and ask what type we are. It's his marrow and blood, after all. He should keep track of this stuff.

"Budweiser," is his answer.

When I made it home last year, I was hooked up to an IV in our living room for four hours a day. My wife and daughters had to steel themselves to connect and disconnect me from the tubes. I took a zillion drugs, felt crappy and wasn't looking forward to a winter of discontent. I'm still not looking forward to winter, but I thankfully am looking at a lot of that previous life in the rearview mirror.

Sure, I'm still on nine different pills per day and that wacky fight between my brother's marrow and my own still rages on (battlegrounds currently include, in no particular order: my fingernails, my mouth, my eyes and my hair—or lack thereof). I'm told this is a good sign. I have pluck, they say. I'd prefer a Cold War personally, one without Sikorsky-Kalashnikovs.

But I'm looking forward to the future, as opposed to fearing it just a little. Yes, Eckhart Tolle (*http://bit.ly/TV35y1*) would probably sucker-punch me if he knew I wasn't living in "the now." One of my many doctors told me yesterday that I've been through so much, the least she could do was alter my medicine a bit to make it easier. I responded that others have had it much worse than me, trying to sound cavalier. When she softly replied, "Yes, but your struggle has been amazingly tough," I thought the dam was going to burst.

I like to forget the insanity I went through. I like to play make-believe and imagine myself as an ordinary, albeit unemployed, citizen of Metro Detroit. Then I look at Mr. Puffy Face in the mirror and do my best not to cringe. That too, shall pass.

When I originally entered the hospital a year and a half ago, I used my incarceration as an excuse to buy an iPad. Now for my re-birth day, I've snapped up one of those fancy new iPhones. I've used it to find out that bison doesn't work in a bisque and that Buffalo isn't part of the EU.

But we have a steep learning curve, Siri and

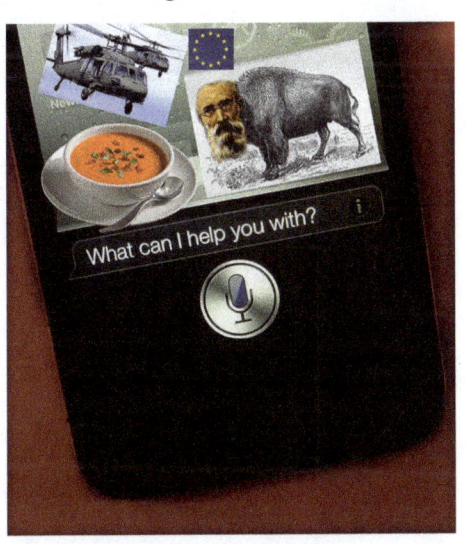

chapter 74 • 199

I. For those of you who don't know, Siri is my phone's voice assistant with attitude. Instead of using my proper email address, thatrodneyguy, Siri called me That Rodney Gut. I guess she thinks I should work on my weight.

But she did get something right. She called me the "Spiritual Wonderbar," bastardizing German and English in one fell swoop. I like it. I think she's on to something. I'm lucky; she could've just as easily referred to me as the Spiritual Wonderbra.

I probably couldn't get away with blaming my brother's blood for that. And I'll bet Queen Victoria's secret wasn't that she was a dude with a small chest. I'll see what Siri has to say on the matter.

CHAPTER 75

# These Poor Corporations

HAVEN'T WE LEARNED over the years that insurance companies know best? Why, just today I received a phone call from my doctor saying Blue Cross wasn't allowing me to take a drug she prescribed. I'm glad that a faceless person in a call center somewhere denied me my medicine. Obviously they have access to all the most advanced medical technology in the world and can judge, far better than my doctor, what's best for me.

Those poor insurance companies. I heard recently that some of their million-dollar executives are having problems sleeping at night. That's unfortunate. Apparently they're worried about what will happen when the Supreme Court tackles a challenge to the Affordable Care Act.

Since being laid off by a CEO who made 37 million dollars earlier this year (*http://bit.ly/TV35y2*), I luckily get to fund my own health insurance and get denied by companies like the appropriately named Humana (*http://bit.ly/TV35y4*). A company with such a pleasant, populace-oriented name can't be all that bad. The guy that rejected my application happily told me over the phone that they don't have to insure people like me until 2014 when the health care act becomes law. Even though he sounded gleeful to inform me, it must have hurt him inside. I feel bad for him, too. Terribly.

Insurance companies have more important worries than accepting people's claims and paying for their coverage. Like worrying about how they can best not comply with the health care act, affectionately known as Obamacare. It must take teams of specialists and lobbyists to think up arguments against giving Americans proper coverage. That would keep me up at night for sure.

Thankfully, insurance companies have advanced far beyond their original intent, to pool risk and spread out the possible harm of something going awry. In those early days, insurance wasn't a for-profit business. Thank God they are today, since they need to employ all those people in call centers who know more than me and my doctor combined.

A man I know in the insurance business told me recently that affordable health care for everybody is just plain un-American. I whole-heartedly agreed. America shouldn't be going around providing care for the homeless or the wretched refuse who can't get a job or are sick. If it was America's job, this phrase would be written on a monument somewhere: **"Give me your tired, your poor, your huddled masses yearning to breathe free, the wretched refuse of your teeming shore. Send these, the homeless, tempest-tossed to me."**

There must be a drug out there that can help the insurance executives sleep better. And if they're lucky, their minions will approve it so they can begin self-medicating. They shouldn't have to go through all this rigmarole in order to fight a national law that benefits the poor and huddled masses.

The executive's worries don't stop at how to destroy national health care; they have to figure out how to make more money for themselves. They are so underpaid compared to the guy who laid me off. Humana's CEO, poor Michael McCallister, has a total accumulated wealth of only slightly over 35 million (*http://bit.ly/TV36lo*). He's gotta find some way to make up that two million deficit if he wants to look respectable around the clubhouse.

There is hope, though, for America's destitute insurance execs. When Aetna's former CEO Ronald Williams left his job this year, he netted 72 million bucks (*http://bit.ly/TV35On*). That could soften his worries of an unthinkable doomsday where everyone in this country is insured.

The World Health Organization ranked America's health care system 37th overall (*http://bit.ly/TV35Ot*). We're right behind the Dominican Republic and Costa Rica. Maybe if we band together and pay the insurance

chapter 75 • 203

executives a little more money, we can raise that standing a notch or two.

Let's all pull together, pool our resources and give them the lifestyle they truly deserve!

CHAPTER 76

# Oh Christmas Tree

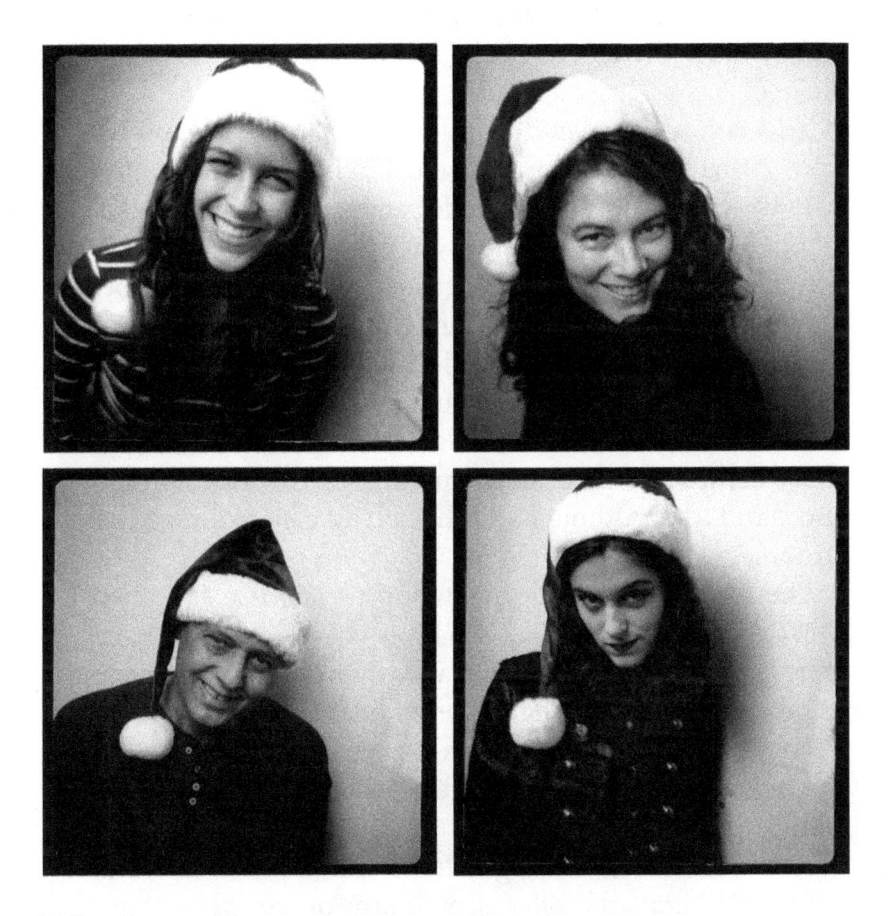

**WELL, THEY UNSTUFFED** me from my cardboard box in the basement and fluffed my limbs, so I guess it's time to make merry again. So far, all I have on me right now are my ever-present lights, which they keep me dressed in all year. The ornaments will come in due course and the presents underneath me, but let me take a few moments to breathe deeply, reflect on the year and sneeze off some of this dust. It's not easy being evergreen.

I noticed something right away. My two younger brothers are also out of their boxes and standing proud around the house. That didn't happen last year; I think the family was still recovering. But now, three of us are stationed around the place and that's always a good sign. Festive, yes, but it tells of the energy here. There's even a Christmas rug in the kitchen. Who the heck has a Christmas rug?

This family has spent the past year distancing themselves from 2010. That year was a plague. 2011 was the cure. There were weeks on end when no one came down into the basement, except the dogs—tended to by a family friend here and there. They traveled all over the place (the family, not the dogs). They visited New York City, Los Angeles, Chicago, Atlanta, Canada, Oregon, Seattle, North Carolina, Kentucky, even seeing some small towns in Ohio. Some quick stops in D.C. and Philly also kept them away from home. It was good to see them out and active again. That's the Curtis family we know and love. Although did they bring me anything? Hello! Ornaments?

Their youngest took up a new sport—lacrosse, it's called. Don't ask me what it is, but she loves it. She also went back to her go-to passions of acting and diving. The kid's amazing. As beautiful as she is long, she even beat her sister onto the Michigan roads and now drives everywhere. We hear a lot of singing going on upstairs and it appears that both of them are taking voice lessons.

The older teen is looking to leave and has been examining small liberal arts colleges, emphasis on *liberal*. Acting has been her livelihood, working behind the scenes as well as in the spotlight. Marching band and leading various progressive groups keep her busy. So much so that when our city mayor said something dumb and hurtful, she organized a protest and ended up on CNN (*http://bit.ly/TV35Ou*), The Huffington Post (*http://huff.to/TV36lv*) and lots of other places too (*http://bit.ly/TV36ly*). If you'll allow a tree pun, she's really branched out!

The mother or wife or whatever role she's playing was always, always busy this year, thank goodness. She takes pictures of everything—weddings, seniors, families, even semi-naked housewives, but we're not supposed to know that. It looks like she has a nice breather for now until the photo season starts up again. So she decided to remodel their home office. I hear dragging and banging and smell painting right up above me lately.

The guy who lives here looks a bit different this year, but he has a smile and that's all that really matters. He hoisted my heavy trunk up the stairs so he seems to be faring rather well. From what I can gather, he's been doing some charity work here and there, writing a lot, too, but mostly just going through the process of getting better. It may seem slow to him, but wow, what a difference a year makes!

Look, I gotta get dressed and spruce up a bit. Get it? Spruce up! So I'll let you go. If the family doesn't say it, I want to wish you a great holiday season from all of us: fake trees, dogs, messy rooms and humans. Have an amazing 2012 and try, unlike us trees, to live *outside of the box*.

CHAPTER **77**

# Tipoff

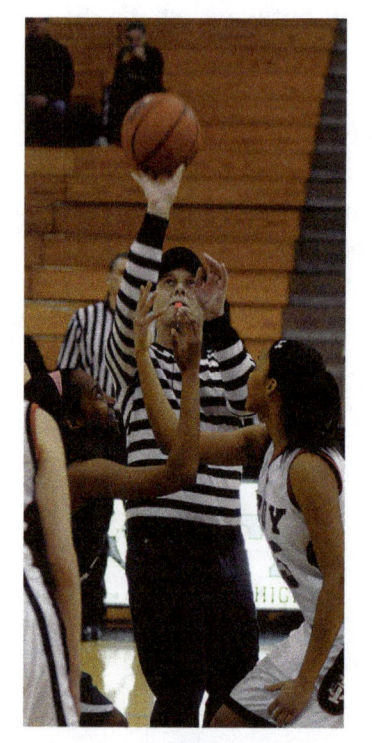

photo by Marci Curtis

I'M NOT SAYING it's because I performed the ceremonial opening tipoff that the Troy Colts destroyed their opponents, 47–28. But I'm not saying it's not.

You can tell by the fierce intensity on the girls' faces that this pretend jump ball was all business. I really didn't quite understand the concept, having only seen people throw out the first pitch in baseball and maybe an honorary coin toss in football. In hockey, do they do the same thing, then get the puck outta there?

But when Taylor's friend asked me to be part of the honorary festivities for Cancer Awareness and said I'd be introduced as someone who beat the Big C, I thought, "Heck, yeah."

Actually, it took a little convincing from Marci, since I didn't feel like being a poster boy. "Sometimes, it's not about you, Rodney," she said. Seeing my daughters smiling and recording me in the stands, I knew she was right.

I was pleasantly surprised by the lady ref who lent me her pink whistle, in honor of her friend who battled breast cancer. But when she coached me on the finer points of ball-tossing, I was certain she was mistaken. Look, I've covered enough basketball games to know they throw it underhand. Sure enough, when the real tip happened, the ref did it the way I remembered.

I may have slam-dunked cancer, but I'm not beyond feeling ridiculous for looking ridiculous. My horizontal stripes notwithstanding.

Each of the girls were playing in honor of someone they knew who were battling or had fought cancer. It was amazing to watch them run onto the court as the announcer read off their loved one's name. And with the way they put a beat down on their opponent, let's just say I wouldn't want to be *any* disease trying to play offense against the Lady Colts.

CHAPTER **78**

# Hello Memories

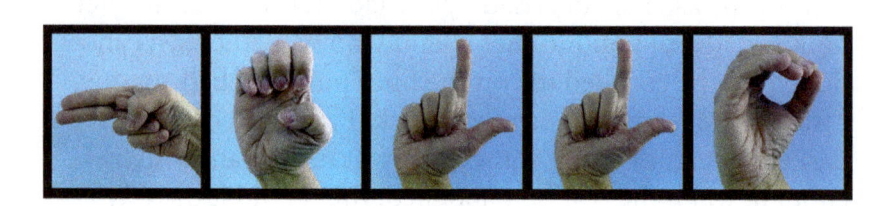

I **LEARNED SIGN** language so I could talk to the cool girls in junior high. They used the one-handed alphabet to communicate behind the teacher's back and since I'd try most anything to fit in, I borrowed a pamphlet from the library and taught myself.

I thank those long-ago girls for teaching me a valuable life skill. Deaf people pretty much scoff when I whip out an H-E-L-L-O, so I just use it to this day as a memory aid. Conversations are fleeting things and if I don't spell something out in my lap, I'm bound to forget it. Especially since the chemo, the transplant medication or the simple truth that I'm aging has robbed me of my once-miraculous memory.

Let me qualify that. My long-term memory is still pretty much what it always has been. I can remember theme songs to long-gone television shows as if I were still sitting in my jammies on my parent's living room floor. Did you know there were two different opening songs to Happy Days (*http://bit.ly/TV35Ox*)?

My cousin Chris was the first to point out my crazy memory. I was telling him stories about the 1960s and 70s while he sat with his mouth literally agape. I shared these memories with him many years ago. I know because I remember remembering. Truthfully, I think my recall is so sharp because I was the youngest of five cousins (six, actually, but I don't like remembering when we lost Russell).

Everything that happened around my brothers and cousins was amazing to me, so it's only natural that I'd remember things like the many different and intricate whiffle ball fields we set up (including the soon-to-be-left field fence we stole from Antioch College during their campus-wide general strike).

That stuff is easy to enshrine in my mind. Some of the stuff I conjure up is just plain weird though. I can barely remember what I saw in some of the world's greatest museums, but I can easily recite the names Greg, Peter, Bobby, Marsha, Jan, Cindy, Mike, Carol, Alice and Sam the Butcher. God, I just did that in a few seconds. I didn't even know that type of critical information was living upstairs. Marsha, Marsha, Marsha.

The information that skips in and out of awareness is more of the short-term variety. If I desperately want to remember something when I get home, I'll spell the first letter with my fingers and hope I remember what it stands for when I walk in from the garage (honest, officer, I couldn't keep both hands on the wheel because I wanted to remember 2% milk and you can't very well do that while making an "M" with your right hand).

My doctors tell me my flash memory will probably come back. All the silly and bizarre transplant complications have made even my word retrieval an issue. Sure, sitting here and typing stuff out gives me time to ponder what exact phrase I'm searching for. As an example, I'm not at all certain "flash memory" is the proper terminology, but give me a pass on that one, please.

I can live with a sparky recollection of immediate things. Some may argue that I could live without the Brady Bunch characters on their tic-tac-toe board in my head as well. But I had a killer ending to this train of thought and I think I lost it when I uncurled my fingers and began typing.

That's my excuse and I'm... umm ...

CHAPTER **79**

# Sweet Dreams

I **WAKE IN** the morning, early, sub-sunrise, smiling in my head and gut. Just returning home from a strange nighttime workshop of the mind. My ladies are asleep, but I can't wait to show them the fluffy hair that's miraculously grown on my head overnight.

If only.

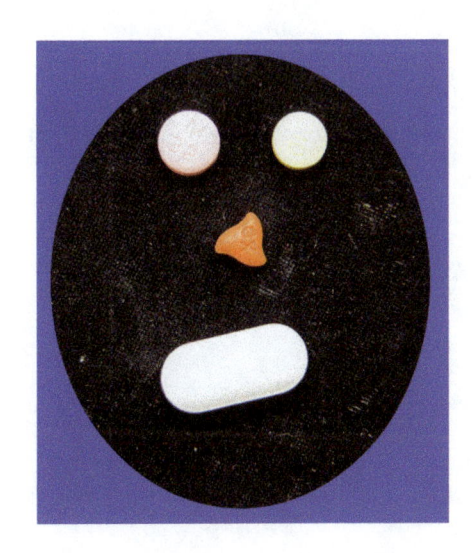

In this dream, my wife and daughters lay all clumped up, sleeping together in the bed and in blanket nests on the floor like they used to create when they were younger. I wake them in my dream; they tiredly stroke my hair to see how it's grown. They're all excited for me. The clock is set back—not daylight saving—but years and years; my daughters are tiny and fresh and beginning.

Smiling so hard, so bright, I feel it in my gut. An actual smile curves my belly. Still smiling as consciousness returns, the deep ache in my void feeling oh so good. I reach up and touch to see if it's possible. Nope, still bald. But boy, the smile's still shouting.

The moon and Jupiter play games with my psyche as they dance close together in the sky. I take a photo of my morning meds because they stare back at me, pill-eyed. I explode with laughter from my belly.

Maybe I'm still asleep.

CHAPTER **80**

# I Forgot to Write About Our Memory Test

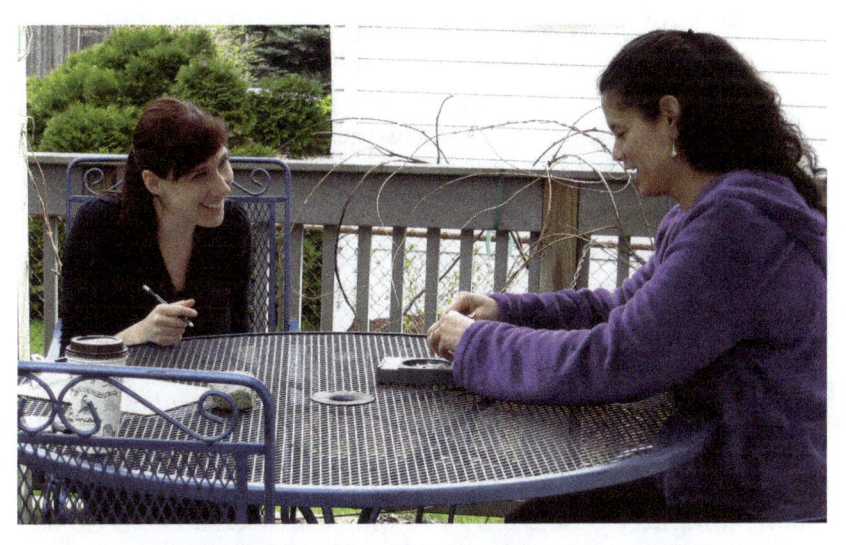

*Researcher Beth Gourley puts Marci through her paces like a rat in a maze, or a wife on a deck.*

**PERHAPS THE VERY** first thing you want to do, when it comes to taking a memory test, is remember that you took a memory test. There might be something else, but I've forgotten it. Marci and I were part of a clinical study a month ago, but I simply forgot about it.

As a bone marrow transplant recipient, my body has played host to many different oddities. Not the least of which seems to be my … my cognitive …

I have word retrieval issues, which isn't a bit scary, being a writer and all. Apparently I'm not alone. So much so, that a team from Eastern Michigan University is testing the phenomenon which—until recently—I've pretty much just chalked up to Chemo Brain.

But no, even though Chemo Brain is real and affects a large portion of cancer patients, apparently those of us who've invited someone else's stem cells to take up residence and play euchre in our bodies have all had memory issues as well.

When I got an email asking if I lived within a few hundred miles of EMU, had had a transplant, wanted to be part of a study, liked getting $25 for being part of a study and have never knowingly engaged in extra-marital affairs with a conch shell, I knew they'd found their patsy.

They wanted to study my "caregiver" too, so Marci and I had "the discussion" about shellfish love vs. un-shellfish love. Yes, she was clean too, but it's always nice to check. So we invited the team over to our house and were a bit nervous until Beth and Natasha showed up.

Beth Gourley, a clinical psychology doctoral student and Natasha Fleming, a master's student in the Clinical Behavioral Program at EMU brought two different testing methods with them, computer-based and good old-fashioned analog, 1970s psychology exams.

**DISCLAIMER:** No electrodes were used in the study of Marci and Rodney, much to my chagrin.

While Beth took me outside to test my memory, Natasha stayed indoors to test Marci. Then we flip-flopped. I won't bore you with all the crazy things we had to do. Some tests included remembering a geometric pattern, repeating a list of random words, tapping buttons in an increasingly complex order (much like that old Simon game (*http://neave.com/simon/*)) and trying to fit together shapes with our non-dominant hands.

I told them I wasn't comfortable hunting for cheese in a maze, so instead they sent me to get some brie at Kroger, but told me to go a different way.

Okay, the shellfish and brie things were made up, but if I were doing a memory test, I'd definitely include them. Maybe that's why I only made it to my sophomore year as a psych major.

The two women couldn't have been more gracious and accommodating. We even had a mutual connection. Turns out our good friend had shot one of their weddings and lives down the street from them. It only took a couple of hours and we have two brand spanking new Target gift cards as our payment.

If you are about to get a bone marrow transplant or have had one in the past few years, Beth would love to come to your place and study you, too. I know that sounds creepy, but you can contact her at bgourley@emich.edu.

**DISCLAIMER**: Never mix shellfish and brie if you expect to live to tell the tale.

CHAPTER **81**

# Spring Eternally Hopes

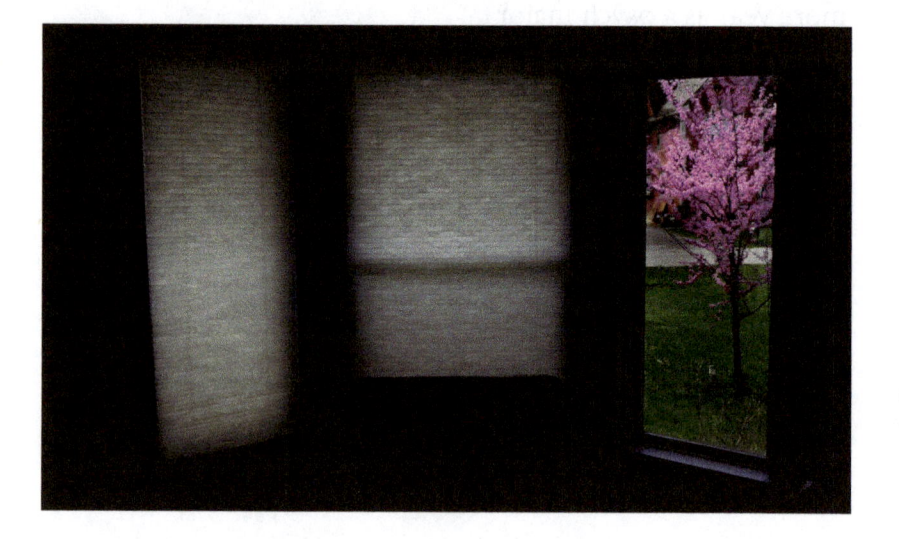

**I SOMETIMES SIT** staring outside, wondering what became of spring, or the fake, funny, vernal tease we had a month ago. It was an enjoyable prelude to things that will come. I've taken it as an allegory for my current, present, now.

The purple tree out front has been holding onto its blooms for what seems like a month or more. Frozen in mid-transformation, it's a cryogenic specimen of life waiting to spring eternal. For some artistic, mythic reason it has paused in its most beautiful and elegant form.

Normally, the temporary swing from winter to summer feels fleeting. The rebirth in all living things wants so desperately to spring forth that their foot race to fruition blurs past us. I am honored to watch and enjoy the stop-motion photography taking place all around me.

This may not be a first—this lengthy, prolonged spring—but it's a first for me, sitting in my armchair as witness. I haven't had the space or maybe *the inclination* in the past to sit still and see the stopwatch click on and click off.

Buds and bulbs push forth from me too. And as is happening with our climate, so too do the fits and starts keep me guessing. But it progresses nonetheless. Hope springs eternal and spring eternally hopes.

CHAPTER **82**

# These Moments

I WANT TO remember these moments. These subtle, daily moments that have come to represent my not-totally-healed self. I fear forgetting them on my onward march toward wholeness.

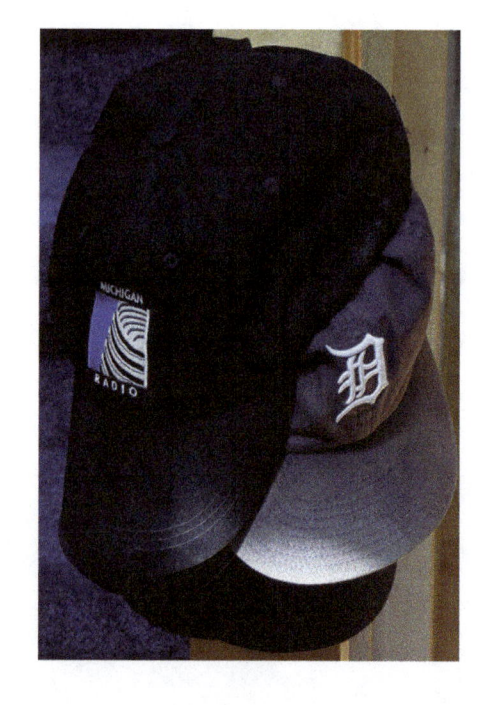

Being shy of my baldness, the myriad stacks of caps that sprout around the house serve as my one consolation to suburban sprawl. When my wife or daughters leave things out and about in the common areas of the house, I'm offended. When I do, it's purpose-driven. Of all the things I hope to remember, I'd like to forget that double standard.

I'd like to remember my pill pile that I visit every morning and evening. Several of them I take because I'm taking several others of them.

I met the lovely Hope yesterday and realized I need to be thankful for littler things. The wonderful young Amal ("Hope" in Arabic) hasn't found a bone marrow match and fears the return of her cancer, as it's done once already. Her *hijab* is a constant companion, just like my baseball hats.

I understood, vaguely and briefly, that I am sometimes too busy rushing toward my ideal self and avoiding the inevitable learning curve that comes from being slowed down by illness beyond my control. Just like losing my job or all the ridiculous things that have jumped in front of me, I want to learn and grow and change from having dealt with them. But in so many ways, I feel like I'm the same old crusty Rodney.

On good days I tell myself that that Rodney guy was pretty cool and ask why I'd want to change him. At bad times I wonder how I've gone through so much without so much as an upward tick on my self-actualization meter. In pushing toward finding a new career and total health, I sometimes seem to forget "the now." And now is loaded with learning.

Moments form steps. One step at a time.

CHAPTER **83**

# There's an App for That

**When I reluctantly** arrived at the emergency room over the weekend, I was convinced my stay would last forever and cost thousands of dollars. I grumbled as I drove down to the ER across from Costco; these visits have cost me so much in the past—time and money.

It was for a ridiculous reason. Remember when they swap out your bone marrow for someone else's, you have to get all your newborn baby shots again? Damn, those babies have it rough. The inoculations hurt and can leave you with flu-like symptoms for days. And they can swell your arm up something fierce.

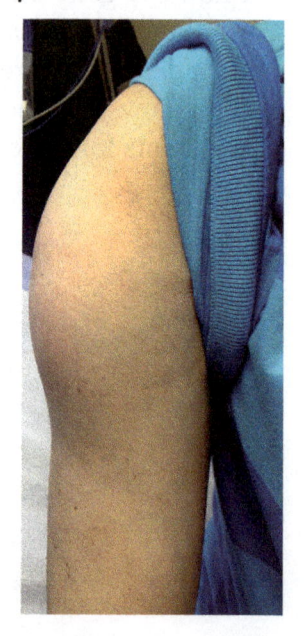

I was fine with just letting nature take its course, but when my bicep got bigger without me pumping iron, my doctors told me to go have it checked out. *Ergh, grumble, moan … okay.*

It turns out, I was the only patient they had and I drew a funny, laid-back doc. He said I was fine and let me know it was a natural reaction. After spending a few minutes chatting he said, "Let me get some pictures."

Okay, a few X-rays and maybe some antihistamines, right? No. Instead, he grabbed my iPhone and snapped some photos using the camera app.

He said, "I'm probably not supposed to do that, but if your arm gets any worse, at least you'll have a record of how it looked before."

I thought that was really smart. A few more questions, a check of my pulse and temperature and I was outta there quicker than a Costco excursion across the street.

I chuckled all the way home. Much more fun than grumbling.

CHAPTER **84**

# If Only I Were a Poet

WATERING THE BARE patches of lawn, dug up by dogs or withered by neglect, a hummingbird drops by.

If only I were a poet, I could describe the feeling, the sense.

Old, busted nozzle, constantly turned to ON, barely useful years ago. Spraying water every which way, some even onto the intended grass.

The main arc—the most relevant stream—attracts a large flapping bug. First glances deceive; it's a feisty Rufous bird, if my color vision isn't fooling me like always.

Oh, if only.

Several sorties, in and out, back and fro. He/she/it even comes to inspect me. The water stream, though, is far more interesting than a middle-aged suburban man on the brink of awareness.

There's learning to be had, epiphanies to be shocked with. Why a hummingbird? Why me?

"Shut up," it hums, "I'm just thirsty."

If only I were a hummingbird.

CHAPTER **85**

# Relay

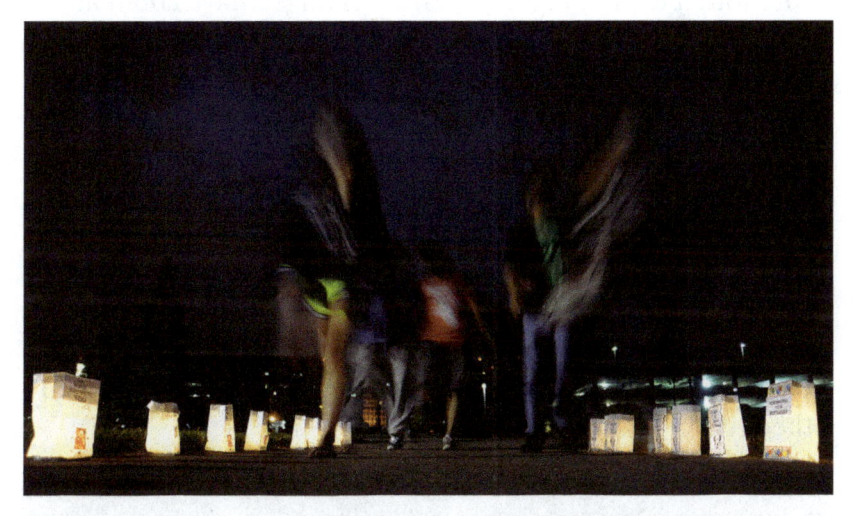

**Late in the evening, Relay For Life walkers blur past lit luminaria bags, honoring those who have battled cancer.**

THE NEW PEDOMETER app on my phone said I walked well over 50 miles at Relay For Life. Even though I'm committed to the cause, that had to be just plain wrong. I think it took into account my evening break, when I drove to Clarkston and back for my cousin's graduation party. I never knew there were aerobic benefits to driving a Prius.

My daughter Taylor is our new hero. She organized her Relay team, "Rodney's Runners," for the second year in a row and made a bunch of money for the American Cancer Society. An emotional speech she gave before the silent luminaria walk last night made all our eyes gush. Just being there, physically being there, was a great way to kick cancer in the rear (view mirror).

Last year, the freak swelling of my heart lining landed me in the hospital right when Relay was going on, throwing the girls back into thoughts of my mortality. This year, nothing was going to stop me from hanging out with Taylor's team, walking laps, kicking around a soccer ball and cracking stupid jokes with them.

It's tough explaining the mess of feelings I have about all this. I met survivors yesterday who talked about food tasting better and animals looking cuter (seriously), but all I care about is my family. Returning them to a sense of normal, everyday stuff matters more than anything else. Yes, this dumb disease has battered and deep-fried us. I have to accept that. But I hate the focus being on me and want my girls to think about regular teen girl stuff (Justin Bieber notwithstanding).

Although there *is* a direct contrast to me wanting the focus to shift anywhere besides me. My family needs to go through this at their own pace. I'd be a total jerk if I forced them to do otherwise.

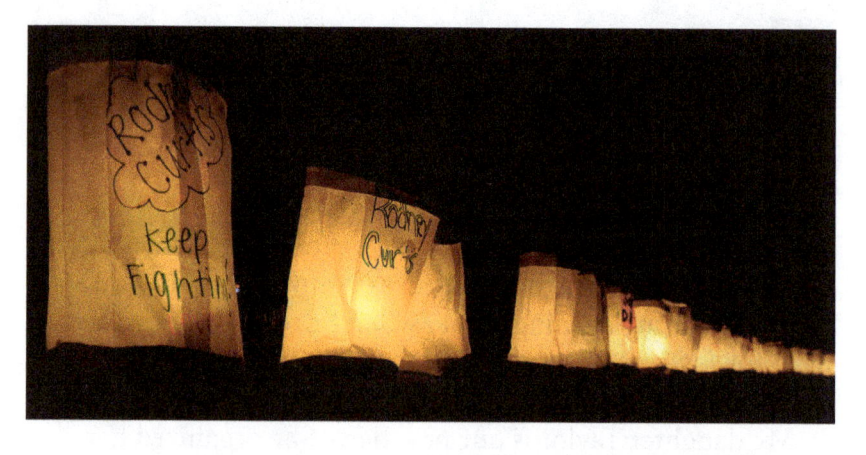

And hey, if you've ever had candles placed in a bag or two with your name on it, honoring your struggle, maybe you know the confusing emotions I feel. If you have, please tell me how I should feel. It's at points like these in my life when I lift up my lens and use the camera as a shield or an artist's palette. Words escape me.

It's my job now to keep the yapping dogs quiet until tomorrow. After the 24-hour event, my exhausted ladies are just beginning to sleep, even though it's after noon on Sunday. My daughter Skye even had a 24-hour band marathon the night before. Charity can be brutal.

CHAPTER **86**

# Graduation Day

**THERE'S A BUZZ** in the house this morning—an energy. Maybe it's the early morning caffeine my sweet wife and I snuck out for. Along the way, we picked up some plants from the megastore and came home to whispers and barking and in-laws and scurrying. I'll take graduation day a thousand times over two years ago.

Two calendar years have flipped, exactly 731 days (counting the leap day) have roared by since the moment the doctor told me 40% of my body was infested. That was a crappy day. Today is preparation, plans, planting, pictures … perfect. You'll allow me the silly alliteration. I'm a bit giddy.

This month has sucked, in recent history. Three Junes ago I was forced out of my profession due to shrinking revenues, yet later on, my company's CEO was paid 37 million to walk away. Then came leukemia, then last year my heart swelled to enormous proportions, thanks to a liter or two of extra heart juice.

Today my heart swells with pride. No trip to the ICU needed for that. Hugs heal.

I love all the whirl around me now. Girls have a way of preparing that boys have never known. Shower, shave, maybe deodorant and we're good. It's a different world for girls on a normal day. Big, special, grand days like this are something altogether different. I don't even know how it's relevant, but last night at midnight, my youngest was trying on my wife's wedding dress.

We can all feel it. Change and new adventure have sent us engraved invitations. Something has clicked for the entire family and it's palpable. Even though my daughter is walking across the dais, in some ways we're all graduating.

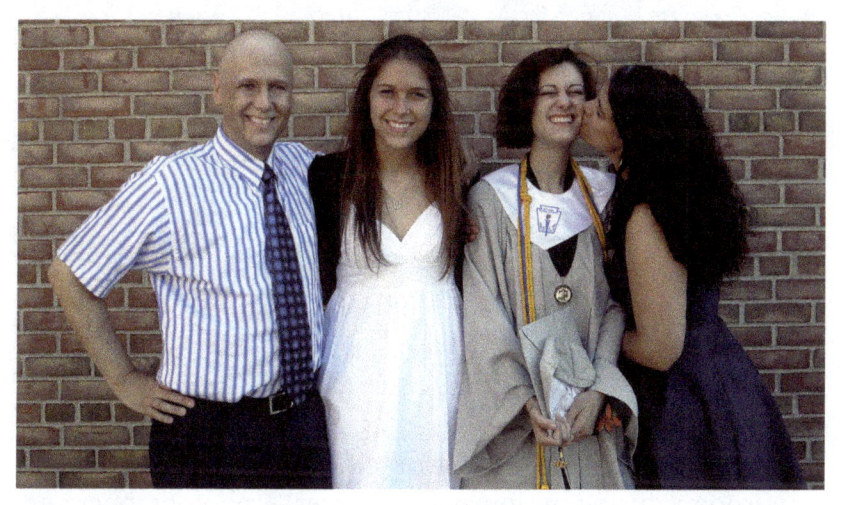

photo by Bill Watson

# About the Author

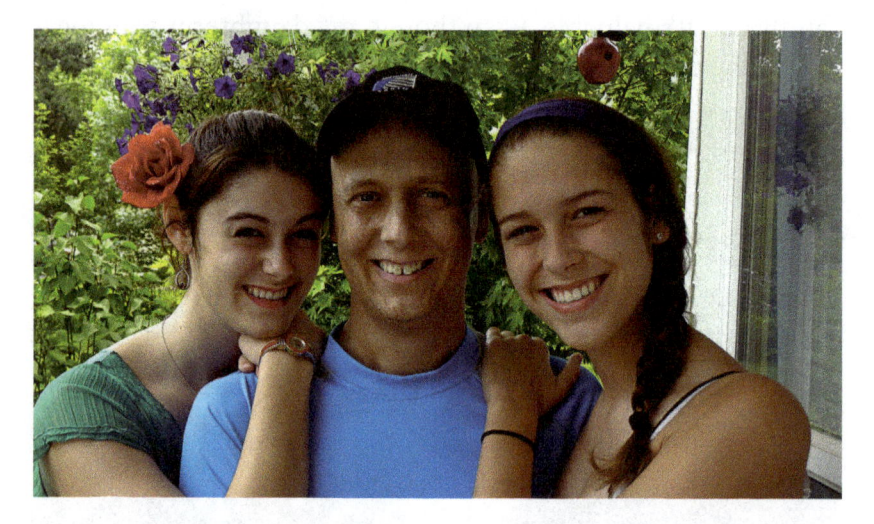

RODNEY CURTIS HAS worked in more than a dozen newsrooms during his journalism career. A photographer and photo editor initially, Rodney also counts being an author, blogger and college professor among his many talents. Rodney brags a lot too, but does so under a third-person guise, so it's okay.

His career has taken him to New Hampshire where he covered presidential primaries, the former Soviet Union, Haiti, all across Europe and through the mean streets and back-alleys of Pleasant Ridge, Michigan, where he was born and raised.

He was twice named Michigan Photo Editor of the Year, has won numerous state and national journalism awards and has really and truly been called one of "Ten Spiritual Sages to

Watch" due to his memoir Spiritual Wanderer. He thinks that's pretty silly though.

His bout with leukemia and his stem cell transplant in 2010 has come to define his current life, although really it's his wife and daughters who've lent all the meaning in the world to his existence. Rodney cares far too much about the Detroit Tigers and iced coffees for his own good.

# Colophon

READ THE SPIRIT Books produces its titles using innovative digital systems that serve the emerging wave of readers who want their books delivered in a wide range of formats—from traditional print to digital readers in many shapes and sizes. This book was produced using this entirely digital process that separates the core content of the book from details of final presentation, a process that increases the flexibility and accessibility of the book's text and images. At the same time, our system ensures a well-designed, easy-to-read experience on all reading platforms, built into the digital data file itself.

David Crumm Media has built a unique production workflow employing a number of XML (Extensible Markup Language) technologies. This workflow, allows us to create a single digital "book" data file that can be delivered quickly in all formats from traditionally bound print-on-paper to nearly any digital reader you care to choose, including Amazon Kindle®, Apple iBook®, Barnes and Noble Nook® and other devices that support the ePub and PDF digital book formats.

And due to the efficient "print-on-demand" process we use for printed books, we invite you to visit us online to learn more about opportunities to order quantities of this book with the possibility of personalizing a "group read" for your organization or congregation by putting your organizations logo and name on the cover of the copies you order. You can even add your own introductory pages to this book for your church or organization.

During production, we use Adobe InDesign®, <Oxygen/>® XML Editor and Microsoft Word® along with custom tools built in-house.

The print edition is set in Minion Pro and Avenir Next.

Cover art and Design by Rick Nease: www.RickNeaseArt.com.

Copy editing and XML styling by Dmitri Barvinok.

Digital encoding and print layout by John Hile.

We would like to thank our copy editors—Dmitri Barvinok, Celeste Dykas and Skye Curtis—who had to endure several Rodneyisms per page and mostly refrained from tearing their hair out until they looked like Rodney, himself. They obviously didn't copy edit that last sentence.

If you enjoyed this book, you may also enjoy

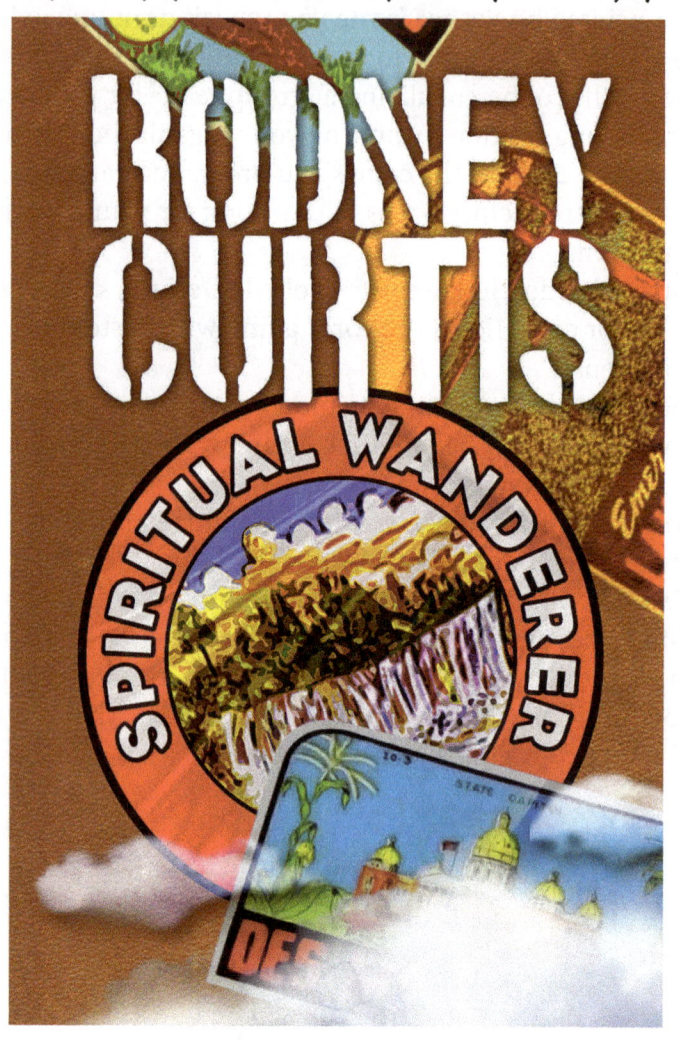

"He's a little bit of Dave Barry, David Sedaris and that fun quirky guy you met on an airplane once all rolled into one." —*from a review on Amazon.com*

*http://www.SpiritualWanderer.com*
*ISBN: 978-1-934879-07-8*

If you enjoyed this book, you may also enjoy

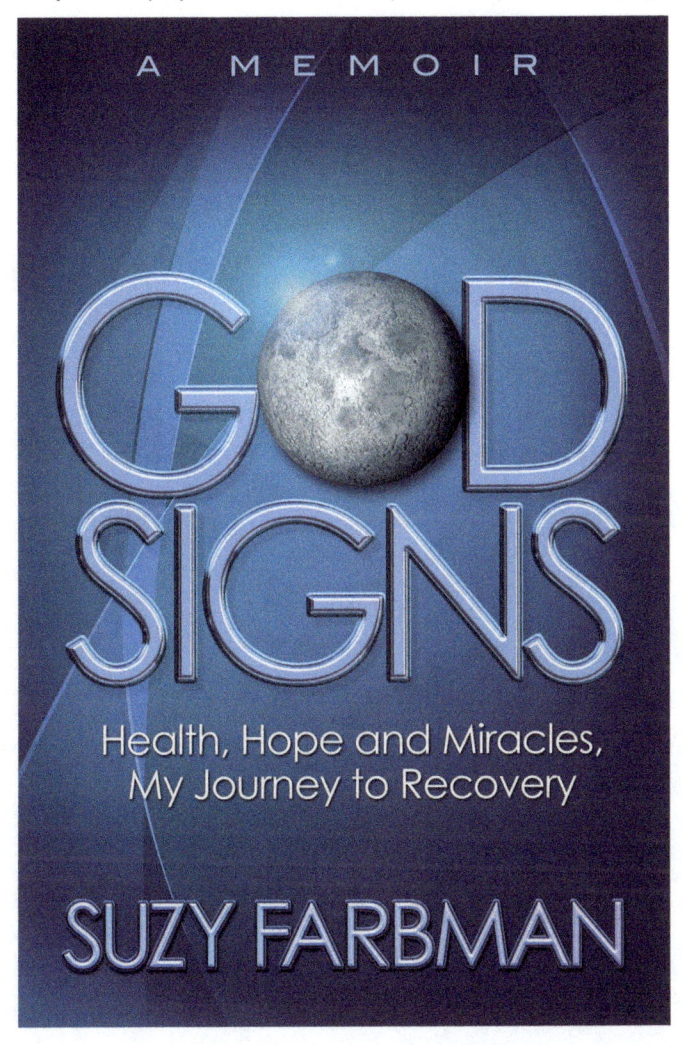

## A MEMOIR
# GOD SIGNS
### Health, Hope and Miracles, My Journey to Recovery
## SUZY FARBMAN

Suzy Farbman has entertained millions of readers throughout her career as a writer. You're in the hands of a wise, often funny and startlingly honest friend in the pages of her books.

*http://www.GodsignsBook.com*

*ISBN: 978-1-934879-58-0*

If you enjoyed this book, you may also enjoy

## A GUIDE FOR CAREGIVERS

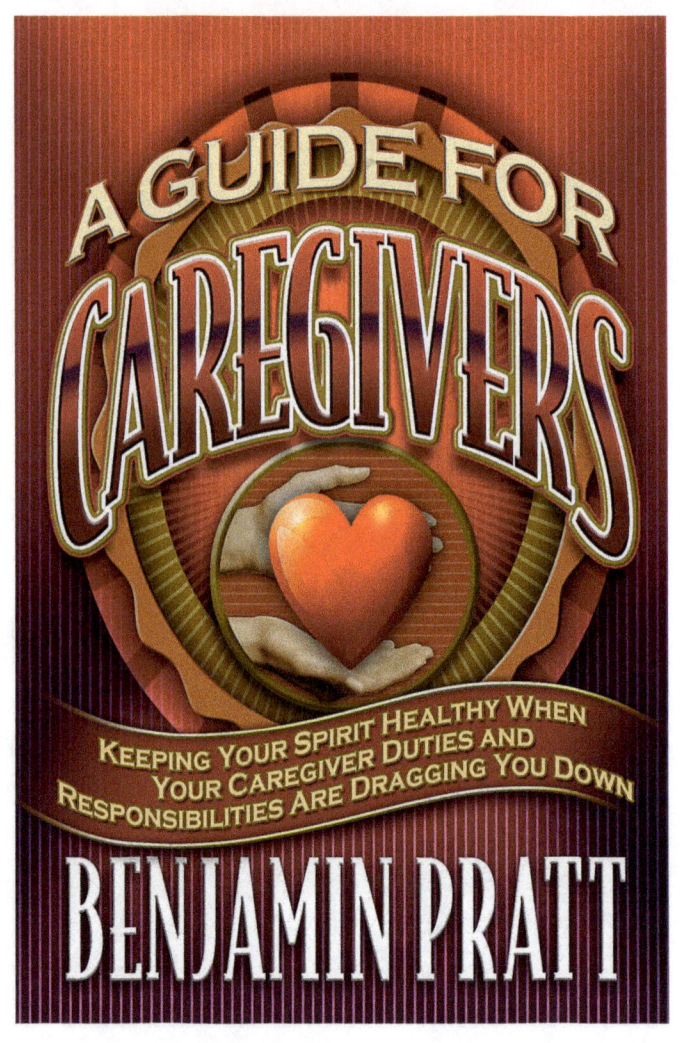

**KEEPING YOUR SPIRIT HEALTHY WHEN YOUR CAREGIVER DUTIES AND RESPONSIBILITIES ARE DRAGGING YOU DOWN**

### BENJAMIN PRATT

In one out of three households, someone is a caregiver: women and men who give of body, mind and soul to care for the well being of others. They need daily, practical help in reviving their spirits and avoiding burnout.

*http://www.GuideForCaregivers.info*

*ISBN: 978-1-934879-27-6*

If you enjoyed this book, you may also enjoy

**Every Day We Are Killing Cancer**
**Heather Jose**

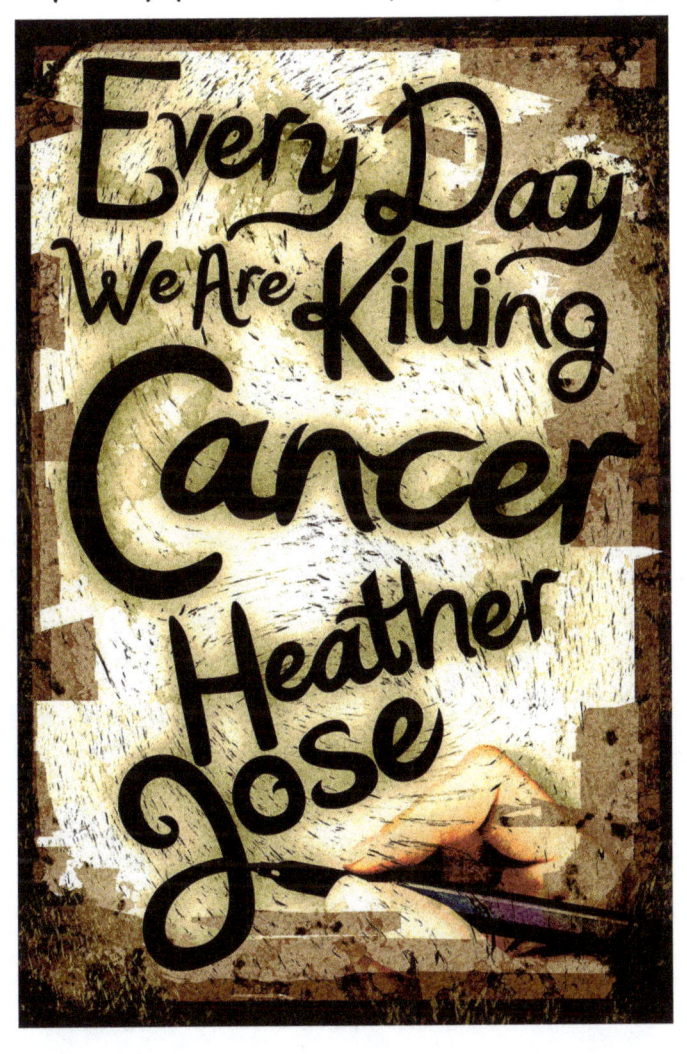

A hand-lettered sign, "We are killing cancer every day," traveled with the family on a long journey that ended in success. This is the story that is inspiring cancer thrivers nationwide.

*http://www.EveryDayWeAreKillingCancer.com*
*ISBN: 978-1-934879-76-4*

CPSIA information can be obtained
at www.ICGtesting.com
Printed in the USA
FSHW011054050619
58705FS